D1375748

MANUAL OF

EVIDENCE-BASED

ADMITTING ORDERS

AND THERAPEUTICS

Karen McDonough &
Eric Larson

Fifth Edition

SAUNDERS

ELSEVIER

SAUNDERS
ELSEVIER

1600 John F. Kennedy Blvd.
Ste 1800
Philadelphia, PA 19103-2899

DATE | 14·12·06
ACC. No. | CLASS No.
009570 | 362·110685
McD

MANUAL OF EVIDENCE-BASED ADMITTING ISBN-13: 978-1-4160-3196-3
ORDERS AND THERAPEUTICS ISBN-10: 1-4160-3196-0

Notice

Knowledge and best practice in this field are constantly changing. As new research and experience broaden our knowledge, changes in practice, treatment and drug therapy may become necessary or appropriate. Readers are advised to check the most current information provided (i) on procedures featured or (ii) by the manufacturer of each product to be administered, to verify the recommended dose or formula, the method and duration of administration, and contraindications. It is the responsibility of the practitioner, relying on their own experience and knowledge of the patient, to make diagnoses, to determine dosages and the best treatment for each individual patient, and to take all appropriate safety precautions. To the fullest extent of the law, neither the Publisher nor the Authors assumes any liability for any injury and/or damage to persons or property arising out of or related to any use of the material contained in this book.

Library of Congress Cataloging-in-Publication Data

McDonough, Karen
  Manual of evidence-based admitting orders and therapeutics / Karen McDonough,
Eric Larson.–5th ed.
    p. ; cm.
  Includes index.
  Rev. ed. of: Manual of admitting orders and therapeutics / Eric B. Larson, James P. Willems,
W. Conrad Liles. 4th ed. c2001.
  ISBN 1-4160-3196-0
    1. Hospital care–Handbooks, manuals, etc.   2. Hospitals–Admission and discharge–
Handbooks, manuals, etc.   3. Therapeutics–Handbooks, manuals, etc.   I. McDonough, Karen.
II. Larson, Eric B. Manual of admitting orders and therapeutics.   III. Title.
    [DNLM: 1. Patient Admission–Handbooks.   2. Admitting Department, Hospital–
organization & administration–Handbooks. 3. Therapeutics–Handbooks. WX 39 L334m 2007]

RA972.L28 2007
362.11068′5–dc22 2006044041

Printed in the United States of America

Last digit is the print number: 9   8   7   6   5   4   3   2   1

Contents

Contributors

Author	Topics Written
John K. Amory, M.D. Associate Professor of Medicine University of Washington Medical Center Consultative & Hospital Medicine Program	Hyperosmolar Hyperglycemic State (Hyperosmolar Nonketotic Coma) Adult Diabetic Ketoacidosis
Jennifer A. Best, M.D. Acting Instructor of Medicine Harborview Medical Center Consultative & Hospital Medicine Program	Acute Hepatitis Acute Arthritis Hyperkalemia Hyponatremia
Alice B. Brownstein, M.D. Acting Instructor of Medicine Associate Director, Emergency Services Harborview Medical Center Emergency Department	Safe and Effective Handoffs (with Anneliese Schleyer)
Melissa M. Hagman, M.D. Acting Instructor of Medicine University of Washington Medical Center Consultative & Hospital Medicine Program	Complications of Cirrhosis Bacterial Endocarditis Comfort Care
Nason P. Hamlin, M.D., F.A.C.P. Clinical Associate Professor of Medicine Director, Medicine Consult Service University of Washington Medical Center Consultative & Hospital Medicine Program	Atrial Fibrillation
Kenneth Jarman, Pharm.D. Clinical Assistant Professor of Pharmacy Harborview Medical Center University of Washington School of Pharmacy	Acute Pain Management

Robert Kalus, M.D.
Acting Instructor of Medicine
Associate Director, Emergency Services
Harborview Medical Center
Emergency Department

Cancer, Admit for
Chemotherapy
Seizure

Diane E. Levitan, M.D.
Acting Instructor of Medicine
University of Washington Medical Center
Consultative & Hospital Medicine
Program

Cholecystitis
Cholangitis
Central Line Infection

Karen A. McDonough, M.D.
Assistant Professor of Medicine
Director, Inpatient Hospitalist Service
University of Washington Medical Center
Consultative & Hospital Medicine Program

Aortic Dissection
Delirium
Falls
Hip Fracture
Febrile Neutropenia
Fever in Injection Drug Use
Meningitis
Diabetic Foot Infection
Fever of Unknown Origin
Acute Ischemic Stroke
Alcohol Withdrawal
Nephrolithiasis
Deep Vein Thrombosis and
Pulmonary Embolism
Diabetes Management in
Hospitalized Patients
DVT Prophylaxis
ST-Elevation Myocardial
Infarction (STEMI)
Unstable Angina (UA) and
Non-ST Elevation Myocardial
Infarction (NSTEMI)

Anneliese M. Schleyer, M.D., M.H.A.
Acting Instructor of Medicine
Director, Inpatient Hospitalist Service
Harborview Medical Center
Consultative & Hospital Medicine
Program

Upper Gastrointestinal Bleed
Lower Gastrointestinal Bleed
Pulmonary Tuberculosis
Prevention of Contrast
Nephropathy
Community Acquired
Pneumonia in
Immunocompetent Adults

Effective Discharge Planning
Safe and Effective Handoffs
(with Alice Brownstein)

Mark W. Smith, M.D.
Acting Instructor of Medicine
Harborview Medical Center
Consultative & Hospital Medicine
Program

Inflammatory Bowel Disease
Severe Sepsis and Septic Shock

Erin C. Sutcliffe, M.D.
Acting Instructor of Medicine
Harborview Medical Center
Consultative & Hospital Medicine
Program

Hypertensive Emergency
Acute Pancreatitis
Small Bowel Obstruction
(SBO)
Acute Renal Failure

Hanny Tan, M.D.
Clinical Instructor of Medicine
Harborview Medical Center
Consultative & Hospital Medicine
Program

Congestive Heart Failure
Diverticulitis

Rachel E. Thompson, M.D.
Acting Instructor of Medicine
Director, Medicine Consult Service
Harborview Medical Center
Consultative & Hospital Medicine
Program

Syncope
Osteomyelitis
COPD Exacerbation
Asthma Exacerbation

Christopher J. Wong, M.D.
Acting Instructor of Medicine
University of Washington Medical Center
Consultative & Hospital Medicine
Program

Gastroparesis
Transfusion

Audrey J. Young, M.D.
Acting Instructor of Medicine
Harborview Medical Center
Consultative & Hospital Medicine
Program

Cellulitis
Pyelonephritis

Preface

Writing medical orders is a skill usually taught to third year medical students by junior house staff. During the first days of a medicine or surgery clerkship, the resident typically sits down with the student to demonstrate how he or she writes orders, and the student is expected to do the same. The end result depends on many variables, including the skill and patience of the resident, the demands of clinical work, and the time available for teaching.

It was no doubt such haphazard and inconsistent instruction that prompted a former medical student, Dr. Nicholas Juele, to suggest this manual over 20 years ago. He expressed dismay and regret that there was no text on admitting orders, and felt that a manual could be used by students, residents, practicing physicians, nursing staff and pharmacists to foster more effective communication in medical orders.

At that time, we were astounded by the number of physicians, residents, ward clerks, nurses, and pharmacists with similar concerns. A 1979 review of the medical order writing practices in the teaching hospitals of the University of Washington revealed the lack of a systematic approach, with ambiguous orders and a general lack of concern for this important means of communication.

In the years since the first edition of the *Manual of Admitting Orders and Therapeutics* was published, the practice of medicine, especially hospital medicine, has changed dramatically. But the need for a systematic, careful approach to medical order writing remains, and that may explain the durability and continued popularity of this modest manual. If anything, the increasing complexity of hospital care; the pace, acuity, and costs of caring for our patients; and now the more widely recognized problems of medical errors and patient safety make the need for this manual even greater now than it was when the first edition was published.

Even more importantly, we are on the verge of widespread use of electronic medical records, and a time when Computerized Physician Order Entry (CPOE) will be the new standard of practice. This was unimaginable 30 years ago and only a glimmer of hope when we wrote subsequent editions. Standardized order sets and CPOE offer the opportunity to improve the quality of hospital care by reminding physicians to order the evidence-based interventions proven to impact patient outcomes.

Purpose

This manual presents a guide to medical order writing, illustrated by sample admitting orders for common illnesses requiring hospitalization. Many illnesses once managed in the hospital are now managed in the outpatient setting; this edition focuses on those usually requiring inpatient care in 2006.

The orders are accompanied by the rationale for each order, and for key recommendations, a rating of the evidence supporting it. We hope that the narrative will also provide the reader with insights into patient care and the specific illnesses being discussed. The *Manual of Evidence-Based Admitting Orders* is not a textbook of medicine, however, and there is no substitute for an up-to-date reference and practice guidelines when dealing with an unfamiliar illness.

Fifth Edition

The fifth edition, now titled *Manual of Evidence-Based Admitting Orders*, has been completely rewritten to reflect the major changes we've experienced in hospital medicine. The Hospital Medicine faculty at the University of Washington Medical Center and its sister institution, Harborview

Medical Center, reviewed current practice, evidence, and guidelines to develop sample order sets for common conditions. These can be used as a guide to writing orders for a patient admitted with a given diagnosis, or as a template for developing standardized order sets, either paper-based or electronic.

Drug doses, indications, and side effects were included in previous editions of the book; however, this information changes frequently and is widely available electronically, for example on ePocrates for PDAs or Micromedex online. A current prescribing reference should always be consulted when prescribing unfamiliar drugs.

Acknowledgments

We especially acknowledge the significant contributions of Mickey Eisenberg, M.D. as coauthor of the first two editions, of Conrad Liles, M.D. as coauthor of the third edition, and of James Willems, M.D. as coauthor of the fourth edition. We are very grateful to the Hospital Medicine faculty at the University of Washington Medical Center and Harborview Medical Center for their enormous contribution to this edition.

Introduction

Philosophy of Admit Orders

"The secret of caring for the patient is caring for the patient."
FRANCIS W. PEABODY, M.D.
The Care of the Patient, 1927

Dr. Peabody's famous statement is a fitting start to a discussion of admission orders. It reminds us that a good set of orders is, by itself, not sufficient for good medical care. In caring for patients, Dr. Peabody says, "The good physician knows his patients through and through." This is especially true when a patient is sick enough to be hospitalized: The inpatient physician must act as a scientist in diagnosing and treating illness, an educator in communicating with the patient and family, and a leader of the team in working together to provide good hospital care. But a systematic and complete set of admission orders can help the physician achieve all these aims.

Admit orders frame a hospitalization, communicating the patient's diagnosis and the planned interventions, medications, labs and studies. The number of possible interventions has grown exponentially over the last few decades and the length of hospitalization has shrunk, so it is crucial that admit orders are organized and thorough. Each set of orders should contain certain elements. Even experienced physicians often use a mnemonic to help remember all of these elements, like ADCA VAN DIMLS, the mnemonic we'll use throughout the book. We've added one additional letter to the traditional mnemonic—a final D for "discharge planning," which is now a critical part of the patient's plan of care, even at the time of admission.

The letters in ADCA VAN DIMLS+D stand for:

A   Admit to
D   Diagnosis
C   Condition
A   Allergies
V   Vital signs
A   Activity
N   Nursing orders
D   Diet
I   IV orders
M   Medication orders
L   Lab and other orders
S   Special orders
      +
D   Discharge plannning

The "Elements of Admission Orders" section on page xxiv will review each of these in more detail.

R ules for Effective Order Writing

1. Write legibly. This may seem obvious, but illegible handwriting still leads to many errors and, even more, calls requesting clarification.
2. Date and time every order.
3. Be clear and specific, especially when asking others to do something.
4. Be respectful of other professionals' time and expertise. Don't request every 4 hours postural vital signs or every 2 hours lab draws unless you have a clear reason to do so, and have discussed it with staff. Writing "please" and "thank you" can go a long way.
5. Have a plan in mind when writing your admit orders. This may only be a plan for the next few hours for an unstable patient. Ideally it will also include a general plan for the

hospitalization and discharge. Having a plan in mind helps you to be complete in writing orders and helps nursing and other staff prioritize tasks. Single orders that dribble in over a period of hours are much less effective.

Standardized Order Sets

This framework can also be used in developing standardized order sets for patients with common diagnoses. More and more hospitals are using order sets, either pre-printed on paper or in a computerized physician order entry (CPOE) system, to ensure evidence-based and efficient treatment. This trend is likely to grow as the United States government, insurers, and quality improvement experts are all promoting CPOE as a way of decreasing medical errors and improving the quality of care.

When using standardized order sets, whether from this book, pre-printed, or CPOE, remember that they are just that—standardized, for the "average" patient. Your patient still deserves individualized orders even if you are starting from an order set. With your patient's history and medications in mind, review each order to ensure that there are no contraindications for *your* patient. Individual orders can be deleted if not appropriate for your patient, and additional orders can be written as needed.

Evidence-Based Orders and Rating the Evidence

The orders in this book could be used as a starting point for the development of standardized order sets. Some of our recommended orders are based on strong evidence from large, high-quality, randomized trials. Many, however, are based on small case series, consensus of experts, individual expert opinion, or personal experience. If there is no strong evidence base for management of a certain problem, practice may vary widely across the country.

Authors reviewed available evidence-based guidelines from professional societies, Cochrane reviews, and a focused Medline search when developing orders for each of the admitting diagnoses. Throughout the book, we have attempted to provide the reader with a rating of the evidence for key recommendations, as well as references to available practice guidelines from subspecialty societies and consensus panels. There are many different rating schemes in the current literature, most of which are quite complicated and difficult to remember. For key recommended orders, we've used a simple guide to the level of supporting evidence, the Strength of Recommendation Taxonomy (SORT) developed by the editors of major family practice journals in 2004. They sought to create an easy to understand rating system focused on outcomes important to patients—morbidity, mortality, symptoms, quality of life, and cost—that would help readers understand the level of supporting evidence behind a given recommendation.

Strength of Recommendation Taxonomy

Strength of Recommendation	Definition
A	Recommendation based on consistent and good quality patient-oriented evidence.
B	Recommendation based on inconsistent or limited quality patient-oriented evidence
C	Recommendation based on usual practice, consensus, opinion, disease-oriented evidence, or case series for studies of diagnosis, treatment, prevention of screening.

From Ebell MH, Siwak J, Weiss BD, et al.: Strength of recommendation taxonomy: A patient centered approach to grading evidence in the medical literature. *American Family Physician* 69:548–556, 2004.

Strength of Recommendation Based on a Body of Evidence

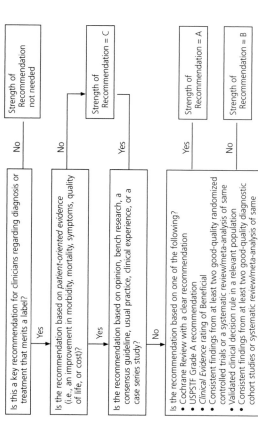

Algorithm for determining the strength of a recommendation based on a body of evidence (applies to clinical recommendations regarding diagnosis, treatment, prevention, or screening). While this algorithm provides a general guideline, authors and editors may adjust the strength of recommendation based on the benefits, harms, and costs of the intervention being recommended. (USPSTF = U.S. Preventive Services Task Force)

Elements of Admission Orders

Here we'll review each element of admission orders in more detail, in the same format we will use throughout the book.

A   Admit to:

This order should specify the attending physician, team or service name, residents, and the pager number for the primary contact on the medical team. It should also specify the type of nursing unit, for example: ICU, telemetry, surgery ward.

The intensity of care provided by a general medicine, telemetry, or step-down unit varies significantly from hospital to hospital. At some hospitals, patients requiring high flow oxygen are routinely cared for in the ICU, while at others, 100% oxygen by face mask is given on the medicine floor with careful supervision. If you are unsure what unit to request, a discussion with the nursing supervisor or charge nurses can ensure your patient receives the optimal level of nursing care.

Example:

Admit to: Medicine ward, attending Dr. Larson, Medicine B. Senior resident Dr. William, intern Dr. Jones, pager 360-4225

D   Diagnosis:

The admission diagnosis is the primary reason for this hospitalization and should be as specific as possible. Complications of the primary diagnosis should also be included. Other diagnoses, acute or chronic, that will significantly affect the patient's inpatient care may also be included in this order, to ensure nursing and other staff are aware of them. Documentation of all diagnoses affecting inpatient care, in the orders, progress notes, or discharge summary, can help ensure appropriate billing.

Example:
Diagnosis: Partial small bowel obstruction, hyponatremia, volume depletion, severe coronary artery disease

C **Condition:**
The condition is your initial impression of the severity of the patient's illness. Some hospitals have a predetermined list of options for admission condition. Patients admitted to the floor with minor illness or anticipated short stays are in "good" or "satisfactory" condition, while those with more severe illness are in "fair" or "serious" condition. Almost all patients admitted to the ICU are in "critical" condition, and patients admitted for comfort care only, for whom death is anticipated, may be in "terminal" condition.
Example:
Condition: serious

A **Allergies and Adverse Reactions:**
List all drug allergies and reactions, including the type of reaction if known. This will be noted in the pharmacy and other records, and new medications will be cross-checked against known allergies. Latex allergy should also be noted in the admit orders, as it may necessitate special nursing procedures and equipment. Finally, major food allergies and adverse reactions, such as peanut allergy, should also be noted here or in the "diet" section.
Example:
Allergies: Penicillin and cephalexin cause rash, codeine causes nausea

V **Vital Signs:**
Most hospital units have a routine schedule for vital signs. For a general medical-surgical floor, the schedule is often on admit and then, if normal, once every 8 hours thereafter. Units providing a higher level of care check vital signs more frequently, as often as

every 15 minutes on initial admission to the ICU. If your patient needs vital signs more frequently than unit routine, specify how frequently they should be checked and for what duration. Remember that very frequent vital signs consume nursing time, and only order them when needed for good patient care.

If postural vital signs or daily weights are needed to help in assessing volume status, they should also be ordered here. The patient's intake and output may also help in assessing volume status and are usually accurate in the ICU patient and the patient taking nothing by mouth. But in ward patients who are eating or using the bathroom independently, intake and output are frequently inaccurate and daily weight (on a consistent scale) is more helpful in assessing net volume loss or gain.

Finally, as patients improve, they may need vital signs *less* frequently than unit routine. You may wish to order "no vital signs between 11 PM and 6 AM" for patients who are stable and are having difficulty with sleep or delirium.

Example:

Vitals: Every 2 hours x 3, then every 4 hours if stable. Please check postural HR and BP in AM, and document intake and output. Daily weight please.

A   Activity:

If there are no restrictions on activity, it is "ad lib," from the Latin *ad libitum*, meaning freely. Activity may be limited because of injury or surgery, for example "touch toe weight bearing R leg" or "no lifting." It may also be limited by the severity of illness or the concern for falls. Patients, especially the elderly, become deconditioned very quickly when confined to bed, so "bedrest" should be prescribed only for ICU or very unstable patients. If falls are a concern, "fall precautions," "out of bed with assistance," and "ambulate with assistance" are all appropriate orders. To ensure frail patients get up safely, you can order "up to chairs for all meals, with assistance" or "please ambulate with assistance daily."

Patients with IV lines, NG tubes, Foley catheters, drains, and sometimes even endotracheal tubes can get out of bed with assistance. Remember to involve nursing and physical therapy when you are concerned about immobility or falls. A physical therapy consultation is a good idea for any patient who has had a recent fall or near fall at home, or has an acute illness that could impact his or her ability to walk. A physical therapy consultation can help maintain the patient's strength and help the hospital team plan a safe discharge.

Example:

Activity: Out of bed with assistance

N   Nursing:

Nursing orders cover many aspects of patient care, including:

- Wound care, for acute surgical wounds as well as chronic ulcers. Nurses are often skilled in choosing from the wide array of wound care products and techniques now available. If the floor nurse is unsure how to manage a wound, wound specialists (often nurses with additional training) are available at many hospitals for consultation.
- Tube and drain care and monitoring. Any tube or drain (e.g., NG tubes, chest tubes, Foley catheters, central lines, surgical and interventional radiology drains) should be noted in the orders and instructions given for further care. NG and chest tubes are typically placed to some type of suction and output monitored. Surgical and interventional radiology drains may need either JP or gravity drainage and

may need to be flushed daily or more often. If you are unsure about how a given tube or drain should be managed, it is usually a good idea to talk to the physician who placed it.

- Oxygen and other respiratory care. Orders for oxygen should include the amount of oxygen to start with and the goal oxygen saturation. For patients with COPD, the usual goal saturation is 89–92%, to avoid the (mostly theoretical) risk of worsening ventilation in someone dependent on hypoxic drive. For most other patients, the goal of oxygen therapy is a saturation over 92%, which corresponds to a PaO_2 of 65 mmHg.

  Nurses may also be asked to educate and assist patients with incentive spirometry and cough and deep breathing exercises, measures to prevent pneumonia in postoperative or bed-bound patients. One or both are typically ordered every 1–2 hours while awake.

  Tracheostomy patients require special care and cleaning, which may be performed by nursing or respiratory therapy.

- Bedside glucose testing. All patients with known diabetes should have capillary blood glucose (CBG) checked 4 times daily when acutely ill, as stress hyperglycemia is common in the hospital and may contribute to adverse outcomes. Patients with hyperglycemia (blood glucose > 126 mg/dL) should also have CBG monitored, as they may have previously undiagnosed diabetes or significant stress hyperglycemia.

- Patient positioning, for example, to keep patient turned on one side or the other if a sacral decubitus ulcer is present.

- Hemoccult testing. Stool hemoccult testing is helpful in patients with anemia and no stool present at the time of rectal exam for testing. Routine hemoccult testing of stool or gastrocult testing of NG aspirate is usually not helpful in the hospital, as positive results may be due to diet or very small amounts of bleeding.

Nursing orders may also request the physician be called for certain vital signs, lab abnormalities, or other events. The vital sign parameters for calling will vary from patient to patient. For example, you may request to be called for a systolic blood pressure below 110 mmHg, or a HR above 110 in a patient with a complicated UTI and a blood pressure of 140/92 in the ER, so that you will be aware of early signs of sepsis. However, you would ask to be called for a much lower SBP, perhaps < 80 mmHg, in the patient with severe congestive heart failure whose baseline blood pressure in clinic is 90/52.

If there is a clinical change or finding that you would be particularly concerned about, such as worsening abdominal pain in a patient with a partial small bowel obstruction, or increasing confusion in a patient with liver failure, you can communicate it to the bedside nurse with an order, a conversation, or preferably both.
Example:
Nursing: NG tube to low intermittent suction. Wet to dry dressing to left heel wound daily
Please call for T > 38.5, SBP > 180 or < 90, HR > 120, or increasing abdominal pain

D **Diet:**
Diet is "general" or "regular" if there are no restrictions and "NPO" if the patient is to have nothing by mouth. Options for patients with specific medical conditions

vary at different hospitals. Common hospital diets are diabetic, renal (low K, low phosphate), low salt, heart healthy or Cardiac (low Na, low fat). Postoperative patients or those with GI illnesses may be on a clear liquid or full liquid diet, and those who have difficulty swallowing may be on a dysphagia or mechanical soft (or blenderized) diet.

Include orders for nutritional supplements like Resource or Ensure in this order. If the patient is being fed with tube feeding via a percutaneous gastrostomy or nasogastric tube, it is also ordered here.

Example:

Diet: NPO

I   **IV:**

The IV order should specify the solution to be given, the rate at which it is to be administered, and any additives you would like. The patient's volume status guides all IV fluid orders: blood pressure, heart rate, weight, jugular venous pressure, BUN, and creatinine can all help in this assessment. Intravenous fluids are generally not prescribed for volume-overloaded patients.

The most commonly prescribed IV fluids solutions are:

- D5 $\frac{1}{2}$ normal saline (D5 $\frac{1}{2}$ NS), which is hyptonic to normal plasma, and is often used as a maintenance fluid, to replace normal electrolyte and free water losses in patients unable to eat normally. A typical, healthy adult requires about 2 L of D5 $\frac{1}{2}$ NS per day as maintenance fluid.
- Normal saline (NS) is an isotonic solution of sodium chloride used for volume and sodium replacement. The amount given depends on the degree of volume depletion and the rate of ongoing fluid losses.

- Lactated Ringers (LR) is an isotonic solution of sodium chloride that also contains small amounts of potassium, calcium, and lactate, which is converted to bicarbonate by the normal liver. It is also used for volume replacement, especially in surgical patients. In medical patients, LR may be used when large volume resuscitation is anticipated (for example, in a patient with DKA), as large volumes of NS can cause a hyperchloremic acidosis. LR should be avoided in patients with renal insufficiency because of its potassium content.

The most common IV fluid additive is potassium chloride (KCl). Twenty meq/L is often added to maintenance IV fluid to replace potassium losses. Avoid adding KCl to IV fluids for patients who are not hypokalemic, those who have renal failure, and those who will be receiving lots of fluid, to prevent iatrogenic hyperkalemia.

The infusion rate is determined by the degree of volume depletion (if any) and the rate of ongoing fluid losses. For patients now volume replete but unable to eat or drink, the rate of maintenance IV fluid (typically D5 $\frac{1}{2}$ NS) varies. Normal losses of free water may be accentuated in acute illness, for example by diarrhea, vomiting, fever, or mechanical ventilation. Most adults require about 2 L per day, but those with higher insensible losses may need more. An order to "heplock IV when patient tolerating PO well" can also be included. For patients with volume depletion, isotonic fluid is given rapidly (typically 1–2 L over the first hour), and then at a slower rate until volume is repleted. Volume resuscitation with NS or LR should be written with a limit to avoid iatrogenic volume overload, for example,

"NS at 250 cc/hour for 8 hours then call me to reassess, please."

An order to "Heplock" means keep an IV in but no IV fluids running.

Example:
IV: NS at 200 cc per hour for 2 L then call physician to reassess

M   Medications:

Medications are a frequent source of confusion and errors in the hospital. Before writing for outpatient medications, review the most recent available medication list with the patient or family to ensure it is correct. As you order new medications in the hospital, check to make sure there are no major interactions with the outpatient list. Also review an up-to-date drug reference, such as Micromedex or ePocrates, when prescribing any unfamiliar medication.

Some outpatient medications should be reconsidered when a patient is in the hospital. Some examples: metformin is contraindicated in patients with hypoxia, heart failure, renal insufficiency, or liver disease. In general, oral diabetes medications should be held if the patient cannot eat normally. Alendronate should not be given unless the patient can drink a full glass of water and sit bolt upright for an hour after the dose. Estrogen and selective estrogen receptor modulators markedly increase the risk of DVT, and the risk persists for weeks after the medication is stopped. Aspirin and clopidogrel are usually stopped in patients with or at significant risk for bleeding.

Other outpatient medications must be continued to avoid complications such as benzodiazepine withdrawal, rebound hypertension with clonidine withdrawal, or ischemia with beta-blocker withdrawal.

For each medication, the full name (preferably the generic name, which is less likely to cause confusion), dose, route of administration, and frequency should be included in the order. Beware of the following unsafe medication orders:

- "g," which can be mistaken for "mg" and should be "mcg" or micrograms.
- "U" for units, which can be mistaken for an additional zero. Write out units.
- You should include a leading zero before a decimal point. .5 mg could be mistaken for 5 mg, but not if it has a leading zero: 0.5 mg.
- Don't include a trailing zero. 5.0 mg could be mistaken for 50 mg. Write 5 mg with no trailing zero.

You may also include orders for "as needed," or prn, medications the patient is likely to require. In addition to medication, dose, route, and frequency, these orders should include the reason the medication should be given. Avoid the practice of indiscriminately ordering a list of prn medications for each and every patient to keep from being called by the nursing staff—you may avoid calls but are sure to cause iatrogenic complications. Routine use of common sleeping medications should generally be avoided in the elderly.

Example:
Medications:
Amlodipine 2.5 mg PO qd. Clamp NG for 30 minutes after dose
Ranitidine 150 mg IV qd
Morphine sulfate 2–4 mg IV q 2 hours prn abdominal pain. Call for inadequate pain relief

L   Labs and Studies:
Order labs needed for the next 24 hours and labs to be done every day if clearly needed. In general, routine

daily labs are probably overused in the hospital. A daily CBC is reasonable for very ill patients, those suspected of bleeding, those with infection and elevated white blood count, and patients on heparin (who are at risk for bleeding and thrombocytopenia). A daily Chem 7 should be ordered for most patients on IV fluids, IV diuretics, and those with significant abnormalities on their initial lab. A daily INR should be ordered for most patients on Coumadin, as drug interactions and illness can affect anticoagulation. Daily ionized calcium and phosphate levels are not needed for most general medical patients, nor are daily liver function tests.

Other studies, such as x-rays, ECGs, echos, and CT scans or MRIs, may be ordered here or may require a separate requisition form, depending on your hospital. To ensure the study is paid for by insurers, orders for radiographic and cardiac studies must include the symptom or diagnosis leading to the request.

Example:

Lab: Q AM CBC, Chem 7

Plain films of the abdomen QAM to follow small bowel obstruction

S   **Special Orders and Considerations:**

Some special orders do not fit in other categories and are ordered here. Requests for respiratory therapy, speech pathology, diabetes education, physical therapy, and occupational therapy require physician orders in most hospitals. Physician consultation is usually requested via phone but is sometimes requested with an order.

As you complete your orders, consider likely complications of the patient's illness and therapies and concerning complaints. You may wish to write an order alerting staff to some of these, such as "Call for any bleeding at catheter insertion site" for a patient with a new dialysis catheter, or "Call for nausea or vomiting" in a patient starting tube feeds.

D   Discharge Planning:

The final step in writing admission orders is starting to think about discharge. Although it may seem early, the plan for the hospitalization can often be outlined at admission, needed interventions ordered early, and potential barriers to discharge identified.

Establish the criteria that must be met for the patient to be discharged from the hospital. For our example patient with partial small bowel obstruction and volume depletion, discharge criteria would include: *(1) abdominal pain improved; (2) NG tube out; (3) tolerating PO fluids well;* and, *(4) electrolytes normal.* Tell the patient what criteria will need to be met for discharge, and give the patient, family, and staff a rough estimate of when discharge might be. Ask if the patient and family anticipate any problems after hospitalization.

Also think about what might keep a patient from being discharged in a timely manner. The amount of care and support available at home is often not adequate to meet the patient's post-discharge needs. A social worker or discharge planner should be consulted early if the patient will need home IV medications, complex wound care, or significant assistance or supervision; to ensure family and friend support is adequate; and to problem solve if it is not. Discharge planning personnel should also be involved early if discharge to a skilled nursing facility is a possibility, as placement can often take several days.

Home safety is often a concern for elderly or debilitated patients. Physical and therapy consult should be ordered at admission for patients with a recent fall or near fall at home, those with an acute illness that could impair function or gait (such as stroke), and those with a prolonged illness or deconditioning. Occupational therapy can also help if you are worried about the patient's ability to perform ADLs independently.

If you are contemplating outpatient IV therapy after discharge, request long-term IV access as soon as medically appropriate (e.g., after blood cultures clear in a patient with bacteremia). Ensure the patient has funding for home IV therapy—most Medicare patients have coverage for antibiotics administered in an outpatient infusion center but not at home.

Many inpatients would also benefit from post-discharge treatment for substance abuse. Early referral to social work or other available resources is indicated.

Finally, a lack of insurance coverage is a red flag for problems at discharge and thereafter. Patients may be unable to pay for discharge medications or ongoing follow-up, leading to prompt readmission and declining health. Consult with social workers or financial counselors to provide resources for immediate health needs and, hopefully, assist the patient in obtaining long-term health insurance.

Last But Not Least—Your Signature

Each set of admission orders (and every order) should be dated, timed, and signed legibly. Include your pager number so that nurses, pharmacists, and others can contact you with questions.

Safe and Effective Handoffs

Alice Brownstein, M.D. and Anneliese Schleyer, M.D., M.H.A.

Hospitalized patients are often cared for by multiple clinicians over the course of a hospital stay. Recent changes in resident work hours and the rise of hospitalists have increased the number of times that a patient's care is "handed off" to a new physician. With each handoff, important information is lost, contributing to errors and near misses, and challenging high-quality care. To ensure seamless care throughout a patient's hospitalization, the physician team must succinctly and efficiently pass pertinent patient information to one another. All of this information should be handed off in written or electronic form, but important clinical information or anticipated problems should usually be communicated verbally as well.

In this section, we review the critical components of handing off a patient's care using the mnemonic "HANDOFFS."

<u>HANDOFFS</u>
H—Hospital location
A—Allergies/medications
N—Name (age)/number
D—?DNAR/diet/DVT prophylaxis
O—Ongoing medical/surgical problems
F—Facts about this hospitalization
F—Follow-up on. . .
S—Scenarios

To illustrate the use of this mnemonic, we have chosen a typical scenario for a patient who was "handed off" to a new physician the afternoon after being admitted to the hospital.

Mr. X is a 43-year-old male patient admitted to the hospital with a left lower lobe community acquired pneumonia and large effusion. He is homeless and has a history of alcohol abuse and iron deficiency anemia. He takes no medications and has no known drug allergies. At the time that his care is transferred to the covering clinician, his vital signs are temperature 39.2, BP 132/86, HR 92, RR 26, and oxygen saturation is 92%/2 L by nasal cannula. He is oriented to self and place, but not to date. The patient has just undergone a diagnostic and therapeutic thoracentesis that revealed an exudative effusion. Post-procedure chest x-ray shows a small remaining effusion with a large consolidated infiltrate but does not indicate evidence of pneumothorax. The patient tolerated the procedure well.

When handing off the patient's care to the nighttime team, the primary team provided the following information:

H —Hospital Location

3e Hospital, Room 13

A —Allergies and Medications

NKDA
Medications:
Ceftriaxone 1g IV every 24 hours and azithromycin 250 mg IV every 24 hours
Acetaminophen 650 mg PO every 4–6 hours as needed for fever or pain
Thiamine 100 mg PO every day for 3 days
Multivitamin with folate one PO every day
Standard alcohol withdrawal protocol

N —Name (Age)/Number

D —?DNAR/Diet/DVT Prophylaxis

D 1—?DNAR

Full code

A patient's code status is a critical part of the handoff, especially if resuscitation efforts are to be limited. However, code status only addresses interventions provided in the event of cardiopulmonary arrest—"do not attempt resuscitation" is not the same as "do not treat any medical issues that arise overnight." If questions are likely to come up overnight, include information about the overall goals of care in your handoff, such as:

"The patient is DNAR, but would like to continue antibiotics, IV fluids, and other therapies until her family arrives from Japan."

"The patient is DNAR, and the goal is comfort only. No new drugs or treatments unless they are for comfort."

D 2—Diet

Regular diet

Cross covering physicians often get called about a patient's diet: Can it be advanced? Can it be resumed after the procedure done today? Does the patient need to be NPO for tomorrow morning's CT scan or not?

D 3—DVT Prophylaxis

Heparin 5000 units SQ three times per day

O —Ongoing Medical/Surgical Problems

1. *Community acquired pneumonia*
2. *Left-sided parapneumonic effusion*
3. *History of alcohol abuse with withdrawal seizures*
4. *Iron deficiency anemia*

Only problems that are active *or* may impact care overnight should be included in the handoff. For example, a history of coronary artery disease, status post stenting should be included—if the patient develops chest pain overnight, it would be critical for the nighttime team to know this history. But including a history of an appendectomy or seasonal allergic rhinitis is unlikely to impact care, slows down the handoff, and may obscure more important problems.

F —Facts About This Hospitalization

1. *Oxygen saturation 92% on 2 L nasal cannula after thoracentesis*
2. *One peripheral 18 Gauge IV in place, access required*
3. *Status post diagnostic and therapeutic thoracentesis, post-procedure CXR without pneumothorax*
4. *Consultants: none*

When deciding what facts about hospitalization to include, think about what your covering physician might need to know to deal with problems or questions overnight. A recent procedure should be included, as complications may manifest later on.

One of the most common calls a covering physician gets is "The patient's IV fell out—does he need a new one?" Stating whether IV access is needed will save someone else from trying to figure it out from the problem list, medications, or chart.

F —Follow-Up on. . .

Nothing to check overnight

If labs or studies require follow-up overnight, tell the covering physician what you are looking for and what to do with the result. "Follow-up on abdominal CT" is a bad handoff. "Follow-up on abdominal CT—if evidence of diverticular abscess, please consult general surgery" is better.

S —Scenarios

If the patient becomes agitated, evaluate for worsening alcohol withdrawal versus worsening pneumonia/sepsis. Consider repeat CXR.

Many overnight problems can be anticipated—tell the covering physician what you would recommend doing if these problems occur.

Case Follow-Up:

Overnight, Mr. X became agitated and acutely desaturated with an oxygen saturation of 86%/2 L nasal cannula. Temperature 38.7, BP was 158/98, HR 122, RR 32.

The covering physician went to evaluate the patient and noted decreased breath sounds on the left side. Her differential diagnosis included worsening pneumonia, reaccumulation of parapneumonic effusion, and re-expansion pulmonary edema versus pneumothorax secondary to recent thoracentesis. She ordered a stat portable CXR that revealed a large left-sided pneumothorax. A chest tube was placed at the bedside and the patient clinically improved.

Because of information included on the handoff sheet, the covering physician knew that a significant change had occurred. The data in the handoff helped to narrow the differential diagnosis and led to a rapid discovery and treatment of the pneumothorax.

Effective Discharge Planning

Anneliese M. Schleyer, M.D., M.H.A.

Hospital stays are getting shorter, and patients are being discharged "quicker and sicker." With shorter lengths of stay, effective discharge planning is imperative. A little bit of forethought can go a long way in preventing complications and avoiding future hospitalizations. Patients and families, primary care providers (PCPs), social workers, discharge planners, nurses, and therapists all have important roles to play in discharge planning. With the help of this team, inpatient physicians must:

- Establish the goals of the hospitalization.
- Assess the patient's care needs post-discharge, and determine whether these needs can be met in the patient's prior home.
- Establish a plan for outpatient follow-up.
- Ensure that patients and outpatient physicians understand the plans for post-discharge care.

Start discharge planning **EARLY**—the time of admission is not too soon to start. The first questions to ask are:

1. **What are the goals of this hospitalization?**
   Establish the goals early and communicate with patients, family, and staff. For example, for a patient admitted with hip fracture, goals would include hip fracture repair and, postoperatively, stable clinical status and oral pain control, then discharge to a skilled nursing facility (SNF) for ongoing rehabilitation.
2. **Where was the patient living before admission, and will his/her post-discharge needs allow him/her to return there?**
   Think about the treatment plan after discharge. If the patient will need IV antibiotics, complex wound care, or rehabilitation therapy, involve a social worker or

discharge planner as soon as possible. Some patients may be able to manage these therapies at home, while others may require temporary SNF placement.

Ask if the patient's prior living arrangement is safe. Is a higher level of ongoing care such as an assisted living facility or SNF required? Consider social/psychiatric factors that may compromise home care, compliance, ability to take pills, substance use, cognitive impairment, and baseline functional status. The patient's primary care physician and family members can provide invaluable information—with the patient's permission, ask them early.

If the patient is homeless, involve social work ASAP and consider respite or day rest centers after discharge. Remember that paying for discharge medications can be difficult for homeless or uninsured patients, and ask a social worker or financial counselor to address this issue as well.

The discharge plan and discharge orders must also address:

Discharge Medications

Discharge medications are a common cause of confusion, errors, and adverse events. Critical steps in prescribing discharge medications are:

- Establish a *complete* outpatient medication list at the time of admission. Verify that patients are actually taking these medications outside of the hospital.
- Review new medications for interactions with existing outpatient medications.
- Discontinue medications that are no longer indicated.

- Plan necessary lab monitoring and follow-up of new medications after discharge.
- Educate the patient about his/her medications. Ensure that instructions are provided in a manner and language that the patient can understand.
- Provide a complete, up-to-date, and accurate medication list to both the patient and the primary care physician at the time of discharge.

The first step in prescribing the correct discharge medications is knowing what medications the patient was taking prior to admission. This list should include all over-the-counter and herbal medications, as they are just as likely to have drug interactions and side effects as prescription medications. If the patient and family do not have an accurate list, pharmacy records or information from the PCP can help.

As new medications are added in the hospital, review their possible interactions with the outpatient medications and adjust as necessary. This is especially important for patients on warfarin; antibiotics, antiarrhythmics, and many other medications can interact with warfarin, potentially putting the patient at risk for serious bleeding.

Some new medications will require follow-up lab monitoring after discharge, such as an INR for a patient started on wafarin, a serum creatinine and potassium for a patient started on an ACE inhibitor, or a weekly CBC and chemistry panel for a patient discharged on IV antibiotics. Arrangements for lab monitoring should be made prior to discharge, *including* identification of the physician who will follow up on the results.

Patient education about medications should start early, especially if the patient is starting anticoagulants, insulin, inhalers, or will be on IV medications at home. Hospital pharmacists, nurses, and doctors can all teach patients about medications—just make sure that *someone* does it. If a patient's family will be helping with medications after discharge, they should be included in teaching sessions. If a patient has had trouble taking medications, consider a medi-set or a home nursing visit to review medications and assess how they are being taken.

Patient education should include side effects of new drugs and when and whom to call if they occur. For example, tell the patient, "rash is common but call 9-1-1 immediately if you have problems breathing." "Rash is common but, if minor, finish the antibiotics anyway." Give patients specific parameters/tips for taking medications.

On the day of discharge, review the outpatient and inpatient medication lists as you order the discharge medications. Specifically tell the patient which home medications are being discontinued. Both the patient and the outpatient physician should receive a correct, complete, and up-to-date medication list at the time of discharge.

Discharge Diet

If the patient needs a new, special diet (i.e., heart healthy, soft, diabetic), a nutritionist should start teaching early. If a patient has difficulty swallowing, a speech therapist should make recommendations for a specific diet and safe eating practices. Consider the patient's ability to obtain and prepare food. Does this patient need assistance or delivered meals?

Discharge Activity

Many patients can resume their pre-hospital level of activity, but some face new restrictions, which should be outlined in discharge orders and education. For example, a patient who has had a pelvic fracture may be instructed to "weight bear as tolerated on right leg, with walker." Physical and occupational therapists can make recommendations for safe levels of activity, and discharge activity orders should include outpatient physical or occupational therapy as needed. Physical and occupational therapists can also conduct home visits to assess patient safety.

Discharge activity orders should also include any restrictions on driving. Patients should be instructed not to drive if on new or increased doses of narcotics or if they have had seizures. If a patient has been admitted for a neurologic or cardiac problem, you may also caution about driving until clinically stable.

Wound Care and Dressing Changes

Be very specific about the goals of wound care and the type and frequency of dressing changes. Talk to wound care specialists—they have excellent tips and creative solutions for successful wound care and dressing changes. Begin educating the patient about wound care early, with the patient performing the care with the assistance of the nurse. If a patient is not able to perform his own wound care, can a family member or friend help? Does the patient need assistance from a visiting nurse? Can daily dressing changes be done in clinic? Finally, consider other interventions that may promote healing or prevent recurrence of a wound, such as better footwear for a diabetic or a new wheelchair seat pad. Provide patients with all wound care supplies necessary to last them until a scheduled follow-up appointment.

Discharge Follow-Up

At discharge, a clear follow-up plan should be communicated to both the patient and the outpatient physicians. Discuss the plan with the patient's outpatient provider, who can often follow up on most medical issues. If consultants have been involved in the patient's in-hospital care, ask whether subspecialty follow-up is needed and in what time frame. Schedule specialty clinic follow-up appointments prior to discharge if possible. Schedule any lab or radiology studies needed prior to the first follow-up visit.

The patient should understand any specific reasons for calling an emergency helpline, returning to the Emergency Room, or following up in clinic sooner than scheduled.

The Discharge Handoff

At discharge, responsibility for the patient's ongoing care is shifted from the inpatient to the outpatient physicians. Effective communication between the two, whether by phone, fax, or dictation, is crucial. For patients needing early follow-up or a specific intervention, a telephone call is best, with a copy of the discharge summary to follow by mail or fax.

At a minimum, the discharge summary should include:

- Discharge diagnoses.
- Procedures performed.
- In-hospital consultations, including name of consultant and related contact information.
- Results pending at the time of discharge, such as pending TSH or pending final sensitivities for positive blood culture bacteria and who will be responsible for follow-up of results.
- Follow-up "action items" that the outpatient physician needs to act on, such as a follow-up chest CT in 3 months or outpatient referral for physical therapy in addition to final results. These should be clearly outlined and, if crucial, communicated by telephone as well.
- Brief summary of presenting history, exam, and hospital course.
- Accurate discharge medication list, diet, activity, and wound care.
- Follow-up plan.
- Whom to call with questions.

ST-Elevation Myocardial Infarction

ST-elevation myocardial infarction (STEMI) is distinguished from other acute coronary syndromes by:

- The finding of ST elevation or new left bundle branch block on ECG
- The need to immediately consider reperfusion therapy, either with fibrinolytics or percutaneous coronary intervention (PCI)

The decision to treat with fibrinolytics or PCI should be made within 30 minutes of arrival at the emergency department (ED). The availability of immediate PCI, the duration of symptoms prior to arrival, and the patient's clinical status and comorbidities all contribute to this decision, which is complex and is not reviewed in detail here. Interested readers are referred to current guidelines in Antman, et al, 2004.

In general, patients with cardiogenic shock or acute pulmonary edema have very high mortality and should undergo PCI even if transfer to another hospital is required.

For patients with < 12 hours of symptoms, PCI is the preferred therapy if it can be performed within 90 minutes of presentation. Patients without access to PCI should be assessed for contraindications to fibrinolytic therapy, which should be administered if no contraindications are present.

These orders are for a 65-year-old man presenting with 2 hours of chest pain, who was found to have anterior ST elevation and has undergone an urgent cardiac catheterization with stenting of the left anterior descending (LAD).

A Recommendation based on consistent and good quality patient-oriented evidence. **B** Recommendation based on inconsistent or limited quality patient-oriented evidence. **C** Recommendation based on usual practice, consensus, opinion, disease-oriented evidence, or case series for studies of diagnosis, treatment, and prevention of screening.

A dmit to: Coronary Care Unit (CCU)

Most patients with acute STEMI are admitted to the CCU, often after urgent PCI has been performed. At some hospitals, patients who have had successful interventions and are free of chest pain may be admitted to step-down units.

D iagnosis: STEMI

C ondition: Guarded

The mortality of acute myocardial infarction (MI) has decreased from 30% to < 10% in the past 2 decades, but mortality is still substantial.

V ital Signs:

Unit routine
Continuous telemetry monitoring
Most CCUs have well-established routines for vital sign monitoring, starting several times per hour and decreasing if the patient is stable.

A llergies: NKDA

A ctivity: Bedrest

If the patient is stable and without recurrent chest pain, activity can be increased.

N ursing:

O$_2$ 2 L, increase as necessary to maintain oxygen saturation
   > 93%

Guaiac all stools
Check blood glucose before each meal and at bedtime

Low-flow oxygen (i.e., 2 L per nasal cannula) should be given to all patients presenting with chest pain. If inadequate oxygenation is contributing to ischemia, more supplemental oxygen will help.

Because antiplatelet agents and anticoagulants are usually prescribed, patients should be monitored for evidence of bleeding.

Hyperglycemia is associated with worse outcomes in acute coronary syndromes and should be treated if present, especially in patients with complicated courses. ➌

D iet: Heart Healthy Diet

Nutrition consultation for diet teaching prior to discharge

A "heart healthy" diet should be prescribed for patients with coronary artery disease (CAD), both in the hospital and post discharge.

Patients having cardiac catheterization should be kept NPO for 6 hours prior to the procedure.

IV Fluids: NaHCO$_3$ 3 Amps in 1 Liter D5W— Administer 250 mL/h × 1 Hour, then 80 mL/h × 6 Hours, then Saline Lock

Patients with diabetic nephropathy or renal insufficiency having cardiac catheterization should be hydrated to prevent contrast nephropathy. A single-center study found sodium bicarbonate solution to be more effective than saline. Three amps of sodium bicarbonate mixed in 1 L of D5W should be given at 3 mL/kg for 1 hour, then 1 mL/kg for 6 hours after contrast. Intervention for STEMI should not be delayed for fluid administration. ➊

Patients who are stable and able to eat do not require maintenance IV fluids.

Medications:

Aspirin 325 mg PO qd, first now if not already given

Clopidogrel 75 mg PO qd

Metoprolol 50 mg PO q 12 hours—begin in AM. Hold for SBP < 100 mmHg, HR < 50 bpm, and call MD

Eptifibatide 2 μg/kg/min for 18 hours post-stent placement

Enalapril 2.5 mg PO q 12 hours—begin in AM. Hold for SBP < 100 mmHg

Nitroglycerin 0.4 mg sublingual (SL) prn chest pain; may repeat in 5 minutes

Morphine sulfate 1–4 mg IV every 5 minutes prn chest pain, not to exceed 10 mg in 1 hour. Hold for sedation, RR < 10 breaths/min, or SBP < 90 mmHg

All patients with STEMI should receive aspirin on initial evaluation by the paramedics or ED, except in cases of aspirin allergy. **Ⓐ**

Clopidogrel is indicated for this patient because he has had a stent placed. **Ⓐ**

Clopidogrel has more recently been shown to reduce mortality regardless of reperfusion strategy. **Ⓐ**

Beta blockers decrease mortality in acute MI and should be prescribed for all patients except those with asthma, heart block, hypotension, or decompensated heart failure (HF). **Ⓐ**

Angiotensin-converting enzyme inhibitors (ACEIs) substantially reduce mortality in patients with anterior MI, ejection fraction (EF) < 40%, or pulmonary congestion. For these patients, ACEI therapy should be started within the first 24 hours, after clinical stabilization, as long as SBP is > 100 mmHg. **Ⓐ**

An angiotensin receptor blocker (ARB) is an alternative for patients who are intolerant of ACEIs. **Ⓑ**

A GpIIb-IIIa antagonist (e.g., eptifibatide or abciximab) is given to patients having PCI, as a bolus (prior to balloon inflation) followed by an infusion for a period after the procedure. **Ⓐ**

Patients treated with fibrinolytics should not be treated with GpIIb-IIIa antagonists.

Sublingual nitroglycerin can be prescribed for chest pain, but an IV infusion of nitroglycerin should be considered for patients with recurrent pain. Nitrates should be avoided in patients with right ventricular (RV) infarction or severe aortic stenosis. **Ⓑ**

Morphine can provide relief of both pain and anxiety. **Ⓑ**

A statin should be started 24–96 hours after presentation with STEMI to improve lipid profile and, possibly, to stabilize coronary plaque. Two large studies have shown a decrease in recurrent ischemia with the early introduction of high-dose atorvastatin, 80 mg/day (compared with placebo in one study, pravastatin 40 mg/day in the other). Some authorities recommend beginning high-dose atorvastatin rather than lower-dose therapy, titrated to effect on low-density lipoprotein (LDL), for patients with STEMI. **Ⓐ**

Heparin anticoagulation is indicated for some patients with acute MI who have not had revascularization and for patients treated with some fibrinolytic agents. Recommendations for heparin therapy differ by fibrinolytic agent, and a protocol for antithrombotic therapy is typically developed based on the fibrinolytic agent used at a given hospital. *See* Cannon, et al, 2004 for further details.

Hyperglycemia is associated with increased mortality in acute MI and in critically ill patients. Glucose should be controlled in acute MI, especially for those patients with complicated courses. **Ⓑ** *See* Diabetes Management, pp 275–280.

Labs and Diagnostic Studies:

ECG on admit, and for recurrent chest pain; creatine kinase, myocardial bound (CK-MB), troponin now; complete blood

count (CBC), M7, prothrombin time (PT), **partial
thromboplastin time (PTT), total cholesterol, high-density
lipoprotein (HDL) cholesterol now; CK-MB in 8 hours**
CBC with platelets, M7, magnesium qd

The diagnosis of STEMI is made based on compatible
clinical presentation with ST elevation in two contiguous
leads or presumed new left bundle branch block (LBBB).
Because a prompt decision to pursue reperfusion improves
outcomes, a decision should not be delayed while waiting for
the results of the CK and troponin. **Ⓐ**

The troponin assays (troponin I and T) are more sensitive
markers of cardiac injury than CK-MB. Troponin typically
begins to rise 4–6 hours after the onset of symptoms. CK-MB
is more sensitive than troponin early in the course of acute
MI because it rises sooner, but troponin is more sensitive
overall. **Ⓑ**

If anemia is found on CBC, transfusion to a hematocrit of
>30–33% has been associated with decreased mortality in a
retrospective review of patients admitted with MI. **Ⓑ**

Discharge Planning:

Discharge education should include:

- Meeting with a nutritionist about a heart healthy diet
- Advice on smoking cessation, if applicable
- Advice on activity and when it is safe to return to work
  and leisure activities
- A review of medications, many of which may be new; for
  patients with a new stent, include specific advice not to
  stop clopidogrel without talking to the cardiologist

Discharge medications should include:

- A beta blocker
- Aspirin
- An ACEI if left ventricular (LV) dysfunction, anterior MI,
  or inadequate BP control on beta blocker

- A statin
- Clopidogrel for most patients, particularly those treated with a stent

Follow-up should be arranged within 1–2 weeks of discharge.

Special Considerations:

A cardiologist should usually be involved in the care of patients with STEMI.

Unusual complications of acute MI include:

- Cardiogenic shock
- Acute mitral regurgitation
- Heart block, with anterior or inferior MI
- Rupture of ventricular septum or free wall

References

Antman EM, Anbe DT, Armstrong PW, et al: ACC/AHA guidelines for management of patients with ST elevation MI. Executive summary. *J Am Coll Cardiol* 44:671–719, 2004.

Cannon CP, Braunwald E, McCabe CH, et al: Intensive versus moderate lipid lowering with statins after acute coronary syndromes. *N Engl J Med* 350:1495–1504, 2004.

Chen ZM, Jiang LX, Chen YP, et al: Addition of clopidogrel to aspirin in 48,852 patients with acute myocardial infarction. *Lancet* 366:1607–1621, 2005.

Unstable Angina (UA) and Non-ST Elevation Myocardial Infarction (NSTEMI)

The non-ST elevation acute coronary syndromes, UA and NSTEMI, are a continuum of disease and are evaluated and treated similarly. Patients with UA/NSTEMI have new or worsening ischemic symptoms at rest or with minimal exertion.

Patients may or may not have ECG changes. Cardiac enzymes are elevated in NSTEMI and normal in UA, and the two syndromes are often impossible to distinguish at presentation.

However, the distinction between UA/NSTEMI and ST-elevation MI is critical because the latter should be treated with immediate reperfusion therapy.

These orders are for a 52-year-old man with a history of hypertension and tobacco use, who presents with 30 minutes of typical chest pain at rest and no ECG changes.

Admit to: CCU

All patients admitted with UA/NSTEMI must be placed on telemetry with ready access to advanced cardiac life support (ACLS) interventions.

Higher-risk patients should be admitted to the CCU, whereas lower-risk patients can be admitted to a step-down unit.

High risk features include:

- Prolonged (> 20 minutes) or ongoing chest pain at rest
- Pulmonary edema
- Rest angina with ST-depression
- Hypotension
- New bundle branch block
- Sustained ventricular tachycardia
- New or worsening mitral regurgitation or HF
- Elevated serum troponin levels
- Accelerating symptoms in the past 2 days

D iagnosis: UA and NSTEMI

C ondition: Guarded

V ital Signs:

Unit routine
Telemetry monitoring

A llergies: NKDA

A ctivity: Bedrest

If the patient is stable and without recurrent chest pain, activity can be increased.

N ursing:

O_2 **2 L per nasal cannula, increase if needed to maintain oxygen saturation > 93%**
Guaiac all stools
Check blood glucose before each meal and at bedtime
Call for recurrent chest pain, SBP < 100 mmHg or > 180 mmHg, HR < 50 bpm or > 100 bpm

Low-flow oxygen (i.e., 2 L per nasal cannula) should be given to all patients presenting with chest pain. If inadequate oxygenation is contributing to ischemia, more supplemental oxygen will help.

Because antiplatelet agents and anticoagulants are usually prescribed for patients admitted with UA/NSTEMI, patients should be monitored for evidence of bleeding.

Hyperglycemia is associated with worse outcomes in acute coronary syndromes and should be treated. ⓑ

D iet: Heart Healthy Diet

Nutrition consultation for diet teaching prior to discharge

A "heart healthy" diet should be prescribed for patients with CAD, both in the hospital and post discharge.

Patients having cardiac catheterization should be kept NPO for 6 hours prior to the procedure.

IV Fluids: Saline Lock

Patients who are eating do not require IV fluids.

Patients with diabetic nephropathy or renal insufficiency should be hydrated prior to cardiac catheterization, to prevent contrast nephropathy. A single-center study found sodium bicarbonate solution to be more effective than saline. Three amps of sodium bicarbonate mixed in 1 L of D5W should be given at 3 mL/kg in the hour prior to contrast, then 1 mL/kg for 6 hours after contrast. ❶

M edications:

Aspirin 325 mg PO qd, first now if not already given
Clopidogrel 300 mg now then 75 mg PO qd
Enoxaparin 1 mg/kg SQ q 12 hours
Metoprolol 50 mg PO q 12 hours—first dose now. Hold for SBP
    < 100 mmHg, HR < 50 bpm, and call MD
Nitroglycerin 0.4 mg SL prn chest pain; may repeat in 5 minutes
Morphine sulfate 1–4 mg IV q 5 minutes prn chest pain, not to
    exceed 10 mg in 1 hour. Hold for sedation, RR < 10 breaths/
    minute, or SBP < 90 mmHg

All patients with UA/NSTEMI should receive aspirin on initial evaluation by the paramedics or ED, except in cases of aspirin allergy. ❶

Clopidogrel improves outcomes in UA/NSTEMI but should be given only to patients *unlikely* to require coronary artery bypass grafting (CABG) in the next week because it causes increased bleeding with CABG. Clopidogrel should also be withheld from other patients at very high risk of bleeding. **Ⓐ**

Although both unfractionated and low-molecular-weight heparins improve outcome in acute coronary syndromes, low-molecular-weight heparins are now preferred because of ease of administration, a lower incidence of heparin-induced thrombocytopenia, and greater efficacy. **Ⓐ**

The dose of enoxaparin must be adjusted, or unfractionated heparin substituted, for patients with morbid obesity and renal insufficiency. Consultation with a pharmacist is recommended.

Beta blockers should be prescribed for all patients with CAD unless specific contraindications (e.g., bronchospasm, heart block, decompensated HF, hypotension) are present. **Ⓐ**

SL nitroglycerin prn should be available to treat recurrent chest pain. However, if chest pain is ongoing or recurrent, an IV nitroglycerin drip should be considered. Remember that nitrates are contraindicated for patients who have taken a phosphodiesterase inhibitor (e.g., Viagra) in the preceding 24 hours. Nitrates should also be avoided in patients suspected of having RV infarction or severe aortic stenosis because the abrupt decrease in preload caused by nitrates can cause severe hypotension in these patients. **Ⓑ**

Morphine or another parenteral narcotic should be used to treat chest pain not relieved promptly by nitroglycerin.

A statin should be started 24–96 hours after presentation with UA/NSTEMI to improve lipid profile and, possibly, to stabilize coronary plaque. Two large studies have shown a decrease in recurrent ischemia with the early introduction of high-dose atorvastatin, 80 mg/day (compared with placebo in one study, pravastatin 40 mg/day in the other). Some authorities recommend beginning high-dose atorvastatin rather than lower-dose therapy, titrated to effect on LDL, for patients with UA/NSTEMI. **Ⓐ**

In consultation with a cardiologist, a GP IIb/IIIa antagonist (e.g., eptifibatide or abciximab) may be started in high-risk patients, including those for whom a cardiac catheterization and possible intervention is planned.

Fibrinolytic therapy is of no benefit in UA/NSTEMI.

Labs and Diagnostic Studies:

ECG on admit, and for recurrent chest pain; CK-MB, troponin I
CBC, M7, PT, PTT, total cholesterol, HDL cholesterol now
CBC with platelets qd

ECG changes (ST depression, T-wave inversion) may be present but are not necessary for diagnosis. If new ST elevation is present on the admit or subsequent ECG, the patient has a STEMI and should be managed differently (*see* ST-Elevation Myocardial Infarction, pp 1–7).

The troponin assays (troponin I and T) are more sensitive markers of cardiac injury than CK-MB. Troponin typically begins to rise 4–6 hours after the onset of symptoms. If the troponin is elevated, a patient has had a NSTEMI rather than unstable angina, in which troponin is normal. Patients with troponin elevations are at substantially higher risk for death and reinfarction than those with normal levels. **Ⓐ**

CK-MB is more sensitive than troponin early in the course of acute MI because it rises sooner, but troponin is more sensitive overall.

A CBC is performed on admission to assess for anemia and infection, both of which may increase the severity and frequency of angina. The CBC should be checked daily during admission to detect bleeding or thrombocytopenia due to antiplatelet and anticoagulant drugs. **Ⓒ**

Discharge Planning:

The length of hospitalization will vary based on the patient's response to initial medical therapy and any interventions performed during the stay.

Prior to discharge, patients should be clinically stable and able to ambulate without chest pain. Patients with ischemia refractory to medical management and patients at high risk of death and reinfarction should undergo catheterization and revascularization as indicated prior to discharge. A cardiologist should be consulted to assist with risk assessment and management.

The appropriate timing of cardiac intervention is less certain for other patients. Some studies support an "early invasive" strategy for patients with UA/NSTEMI, with catheterization within 4–48 hours of hospital admission. Others support a more selective approach to early catheterization. Again, consultation with a cardiologist is indicated to assist with these decisions.

Discharge education should include:

- Meeting with a nutritionist about a heart healthy diet
- Advice on smoking cessation, if applicable
- Advice on activity and when it is safe to return to work and leisure activities
- A review of medications, many of which may be new; for patients with a new stent, include specific advice not to stop clopidogrel without talking to the cardiologist

Discharge medications should include:

- A beta blocker
- Aspirin
- A statin
- An ACEI for those with LV dysfunction or inadequate BP control on beta blocker
- For most patients, especially if a stent has been placed, clopidogrel

Follow-up should be arranged within 1 week for higher-risk patients or within 2–4 weeks for those at lower risk.

Special Considerations:

A cardiologist should be consulted for patients diagnosed with unstable angina or NSTEMI to assist with risk stratification and to arrange catheterization as indicated.

References

Braunwald E, Antman EM, Beasley JW, et al: ACC/AHA 2002 guideline update for the management of patients with unstable angina and non–ST-segment elevation myocardial infarction—summary article. *JACC* 40:1366–1374, 2002.

Cannon CP, Braunwald E, McCabe CH, et al: Intensive versus moderate lipid lowering with statins after acute coronary syndromes. *N Engl J Med* 350:1495–1504, 2004.

De Winter RJ, Windhausen F, Cornel JH, et al: Early invasive versus selectively invasive management for acute coronary syndromes. *N Engl J Med* 353:1095–1104, 2005.

Atrial Fibrillation

Atrial fibrillation (a. fib) is increasingly common as the population ages; 8% of patients older than 80 years carry the diagnosis. Many patients are asymptomatic, having had a. fib for an unknown period of time. Others present with palpitations, dyspnea, fatigue, or even ischemia or HF.

The risk of stroke is substantially increased in a. fib, occurring in 5% of patients per year. When treating a. fib, both control of symptoms and stroke prevention must be addressed.

Admission to the hospital is indicated if ischemia is suspected or if the patient is symptomatic with rapid ventricular response. A. fib may be precipitated by other illnesses requiring admission, such as pneumonia, pulmonary embolism, hyperthyroidism, or alcoholism, and may resolve spontaneously as the precipitating illness is treated.

These orders are for an elderly patient presenting with exercise intolerance who was found to have a. fib at a rate of 130 bpm.

A dmit to: Telemetry

Most patients should be admitted to a telemetry bed for monitoring of HR with initiation of medical therapy. Hemodynamically unstable patients or those with suspected ischemia should be admitted to the ICU/CCU.

D iagnosis: Atrial Fibrillation

C ondition: Guarded

Condition may range from stable to critical, depending on presenting symptoms, vital signs (VS), and comorbid disease.

V ital Signs:

Every 2 hours × 4; then decrease to every 4 hours
Continuous telemetry monitoring

As the HR is controlled, VS may be done less frequently if BP remains stable.

A llergies: Nonsteroidal Anti-Inflammatory Drugs (NSAIDs)

A ctivity: As Tolerated. Teach Patient to Sit at the Side of the Bed for Several Minutes Before Standing

Hemodynamically stable patients can get up in the room, but rapid ventricular response may limit activity tolerance.

Because new cardiac medications can increase the risk of orthostasis and falls, patients should be instructed to stand up slowly and sit down again if they feel at all light headed.

N ursing:

Oxygen at 2 L per nasal cannula if O_2 saturation < 93%

D iet: Heart Healthy Diet

If the patient does not have CAD or hypertension, a general diet can be prescribed.

If cardioversion is anticipated, remember to make the patient NPO for 8 hours prior to the procedure.

IV Fluids: Heplock IV

IV access should be maintained for all patients on telemetry, but IV fluid is not necessary for most patients with a. fib.

M edications:

Metoprolol 5 mg IV over 2–3 minutes; if HR > 100 bpm and SBP > 100 mmHg, repeat every 5 minutes × 2, to a maximum of 15 mg

Metoprolol 50 mg PO every 12 hours—begin in 6 hours

Warfarin 5 mg PO tonight; dose of warfarin to be adjusted daily based on PT/international normalized ratio (INR)

Rate control is the initial goal for most patients admitted with a. fib. The initial target HR should be 80–100 bpm, then medication should be titrated to control rate with exercise as well as at rest. The usual goal is a HR of 60–80 bpm at rest and up to 115 bpm with moderate exercise. **Ⓒ**

Patients with rapid ventricular response causing HF, myocardial ischemia, or symptomatic hypotension should be treated with immediate cardioversion rather than rate control. **Ⓑ**

Because cardioversion carries a risk of stroke, especially if a. fib has been present for more than 48 hours, emergent cardioversion should be reserved for these very select patients. **C**

Patients with rapid ventricular response are typically treated with IV medications, then quickly transitioned to oral medications. Beta blockers and calcium channel blockers are first-line therapies for most patients. The dose-limiting side effect of both is hypotension, and neither should be given to patients with symptomatic hypotension.

Metoprolol and atenolol have been most consistently effective for controlling rate both at rest and with exercise. Metoprolol is available in an IV form, whereas atenolol is not. An esmolol drip is an option if a very short half-life would be an advantage; for example, in patients at risk for hypotension with treatment. **A**

Atrioventricular (AV) nodal blocking calcium channel blockers (verapamil and diltiazem) are also effective for rate control. **A**

Diltiazem is dosed at 0.25 mg/kg IV over 2 minutes and repeated if HR is not adequately controlled after 15 minutes. When rate is controlled, begin continuous infusion at 5–10 mg/h, titrating as necessary. When stable, convert to four times a day (qid) short-acting diltiazem, then to a long-acting preparation on discharge.

Verapamil is dosed 0.075 mg/kg IV over 2 minutes and repeated if rate is not adequately controlled in 15 minutes. Then begin oral verapamil 80–120 mg PO every 8 hours, converting to a long-acting preparation on discharge.

Digoxin controls HR at rest but not with exercise. It is often ineffective even at rest for a. fib associated with other medical illness. It can be used as the first-line drug for patients with contraindication to more effective drugs but is usually used in addition to another drug, if needed. **B**

In the long term, rate control (with chronic anticoagulation) is as effective as maintenance of sinus rhythm in controlling symptoms for most patients with a. fib. There is no mortality benefit to a rhythm control strategy. Selected patients who remain symptomatic despite rate control may be treated with electrical or pharmacologic cardioversion after a period of anticoagulation. ❹

Anticoagulation for prevention of stroke should be recommended for most patients with a. fib unless they are at very low risk of stroke or have specific contraindications to warfarin (e.g., recent surgery, trauma, thrombocytopenia, or alcoholism). ❹

The elderly derive more benefit from anticoagulation for stroke prevention than younger patients, so warfarin should not be withheld from the elderly simply because of their increased risk for falls.

The CHADS2 scoring system can help estimate the risk of stroke in patients with a. fib. One point is assigned for each of the following:

- Congestive heart failure (CHF)
- Hypertension
- Age $\geq$ 75
- Diabetes
- Two points assigned for a history of stroke or transient ischemic attack (TIA)

Patients with 0 or 1 point are at a low yearly risk of stroke (2–3%), those with 2 or 3 points are at moderate risk (4–6%), and those with 4 or more points are high risk (8–19%). The higher the stroke risk, the more likely the patient is to derive benefit from warfarin. ❹

Warfarin can be started at 5 mg/day and adjusted based on INR, without heparin.

Although the benefit of daily aspirin for stroke prevention is not as large as for warfarin, aspirin should be given if warfarin will not be prescribed. ❹

L abs and Diagnostic Studies:

Admit labs: ECG, Chem 7, CBC, chest x-ray (CXR), CK-MB, troponin, thyroid-stimulating hormone (TSH), serum iron and transferrin saturation

Transthoracic echocardiogram

An ECG is done to confirm the diagnosis of a. fib and to evaluate for ischemia. Cardiac enzymes are done if ischemia is suspected. Chem 7, CBC, TSH, and CXR are done to evaluate for concurrent disease that may have led to a. fib. Hemochromatosis may present with a. fib, so screening iron studies should be done once. Further testing for specific precipitating illnesses is guided by the initial history, exam, and labs. **ⓒ**

All patients with newly diagnosed a. fib should have a transthoracic echocardiogram to evaluate for HF and valvular disease. **ⓒ**

Transesophageal echocardiography may be done to exclude left atrial clot if cardioversion without prior anticoagulation is desirable. If no atrial thrombus is detected, the rate of stroke with cardioversion is similar to that of patients anticoagulated for 3 weeks. **Ⓐ**

D ischarge Planning:

If no other illness is diagnosed, patients with a. fib may be discharged as soon as the HR is controlled.

Most patients should be discharged on warfarin. If available, a pharmacist should be consulted for anticoagulation teaching. Follow-up should be arranged in an anticoagulation clinic or with the primary care physician several days after discharge for an INR check and adjustment of warfarin dose.

S pecial Considerations:

Consider cardiology consultation for any patient with evidence of coexistent cardiac disease and when cardioversion is being considered.

Patients with rapid ventricular response and myocardial ischemia or symptomatic hypotension should be cardioverted emergently.

If the onset of a. fib can be timed with certainty (e.g., a patient on telemetry), electrical or pharmacologic cardioversion can be done within 48 hours with a low risk of stroke. Otherwise, 3 weeks of therapeutic anticoagulation should precede cardioversion, if it is to be attempted.

References

The Atrial Fibrillation Follow-Up Investigation of Rhythm Management (AFFIRM). *N Engl J Med* 347:1825–1833, 2002.

Fuster V, Ryden LE, Asinger RW, et al: ACC/AHA/ESC guidelines for the management of patients with atrial fibrillation. *JACC* 38:1231–1266, 2001.

Medical Progress: Atrial Fibrillation. *N Engl J Med* 344:1067–1078, 2001.

Snow V, Weiss KB, Lefevre M, et al: Management of newly detected atrial fibrillation. A practice guideline from the American Academy of Family Physicians and the American College of Physicians. *Ann Intern Med* 139:1009–1017, 2003.

Congestive Heart Failure

CHF accounts for at least 20% of hospital admissions for patients older than 65 years. Patients present with increasing shortness of breath or edema due to increased filling pressures in the left heart, either from systolic or diastolic dysfunction.

Most patients admitted with CHF have systolic dysfunction confirmed by echocardiography. A minority have normal EF, often with evidence of impaired ventricular relaxation, or diastolic dysfunction. The most common cause of diastolic dysfunction is hypertension, but rare causes of restrictive cardiomyopathy, such as amyloidosis, should be considered for younger patients and nonhypertensive patients. HF with normal EF is usually treated with diuretics and antihypertensives.

These orders are for an 80-year-old man with an acute exacerbation of HF with reduced ejection fracture.

A dmit to: Telemetry Floor

The physical examination (especially VS and evaluation of volume status) will guide triage to the floor or ICU.

Mild CHF, with normal RR, oxygenation, and mild to moderate edema, can usually be managed as an outpatient or on a general medicine floor. Patients with a history of arrhythmias and those who will need aggressive diuresis should be on telemetry because rapid diuresis can cause electrolyte loss and arrhythmias.

Patients with severe HF, manifesting as severe hypoxia, respiratory distress, or hypotension, with or without uncontrolled heart rhythms, valvular disorders, or acute myocardial ischemia, should be admitted to the ICU. **B**

If an underlying cause of HF exists (i.e., MI or ventricular or supraventricular arrhythmias), it must be treated along with HF.

D iagnosis: Congestive Heart Failure

C ondition: Guarded

Stable patients can breathe comfortably with aid of low-flow oxygen after initial ED treatment with IV diuretics and have normal VS.

Guarded patients require more oxygen, have more evidence of volume overload, or have active comorbid conditions.

Critical patients are unstable and require an ICU bed.

V ital Signs

On admit and q 4 hours
Orthostatic BP each morning. Call house officer (HO) for RR
    > 30 breaths/minute, increasing O$_2$ requirement, SBP < 95
    mmHg, urine output (UO) < 100 mL/h

If a patient has mild CHF, q shift vitals may be appropriate. If moderate to severe CHF, then BP, RR, and HR may need to be taken more frequently, from hourly (in the ICU) to q 4 hours. Orthostatic BP should be checked at least once daily to assess effects of diuresis.

A llergies: NKDA

A ctivity: Bedrest with Bathroom Privileges, Up Only with Assistance. Fall Precautions

Bedrest may facilitate diuresis.

Patients undergoing diuresis may be at increased risk for falls because of intravascular volume depletion and vasodilating medications. They should be instructed to sit at the edge of the bed for a few minutes prior to standing.

N ursing:

Daily weights
Strict inputs and outputs (I/Os)
Oxygen as needed based to maintain oxygen saturation > 92%

Strict I/Os can be discontinued once the patient's condition is stable. Daily weights are another means of ensuring adequate diuresis. For patients with substantial volume overload and stable renal function, the goal weight loss should be 1–2 kg/day.

D iet: 2 g Sodium Restriction, Heart Healthy Diet

Nutrition consult for teaching on low-sodium diet

Sodium restriction promotes diuresis and prevents further fluid retention. Dietary indiscretion can cause CHF exacerbation. Patient education about a low-sodium diet is crucial to preventing readmission with CHF. ❸

IV Fluids: Heparin Lock

IV fluids should not be given to patients admitted with CHF because the goal is diuresis of salt and water.

M edications:

Furosemide 80 mg IV now, then 60 mg IV bid
Lisinopril 10 mg PO bid
Digoxin 0.125 mg PO qd
Stop carvedilol while hospitalized

Diuretics are the cornerstone of acute therapy for CHF. The majority of patients will improve with IV diuretics alone. The initial furosemide dose is variable depending on the patient's previous dosage and severity of symptoms. Patients previously treated with furosemide usually require higher dosages than naïve patients. ❸

Alternative loop diuretics are bumetanide or torsemide for patients resistant to furosemide. Loop diuretics can also be given as a continuous infusion, with greater efficacy. ❹

For patients resistant to a loop diuretic alone, chlorothiazide 500 mg or metolazone 2.5 mg can be added to increase UO. However, this combination can lead to severe hypokalemia, so very careful lab monitoring is indicated. ❸

Spironolactone, a potassium-sparing aldosterone antagonist, should be added to the diuretic regimen of patients with current or recent New York Heart Association (NYHA) class IV HF and no hyperkalemia or renal insufficiency. ❹

ACEIs, such as lisinopril, enalapril, or ramipril, should be prescribed for all patients with HF with reduced left ventricular ejection fraction (LVEF) unless they have contraindications (most commonly angioedema, hyperkalemia, cough, or significant renal insufficiency.) **Ⓐ**

ARBs, such as losartan or valsartan, should be prescribed for patients unable to tolerate ACEIs. **Ⓐ**

Digoxin has been shown to improve symptoms and decrease hospitalization in patients with CHF. It should be considered for patients who remain symptomatic despite therapy with an ACEI, beta blocker, and diuretic. **Ⓐ**

A beta blocker (carvedilol, metoprolol XL, or bisoprolol) should be added to the medication regimen of all patients with symptomatic HF *after* they are clinically improved with resolution of volume overload. **Ⓐ**

For patients with severe CHF or cardiogenic shock, continuous infusions of IV vasodilators such as nitroprusside or nesiritide or positive inotropes such as dobutamine or milrinone may be indicated. Cardiology consultation may be appropriate for assistance with management of these drugs. **Ⓑ**

Nesiritide, a vasodilator, was introduced for the treatment of HF several years ago. However, recent studies have shown that it may *increase* mortality in acutely decompensated CHF. Cardiology consultation would be appropriate prior to considering this drug.

For patients with significant pulmonary edema, morphine sulfate 2–4 mg IV decreases anxiety and work of breathing, improving vascular resistance and symptoms. Morphine may be repeated, allowing time for IV diuretics to work. **Ⓑ**

Patients with severe dyspnea and pulmonary edema should also be treated with topical or IV nitrates (e.g., nitroglycerin paste 2 inches to chest wall) to provide vasodilation and improve symptoms. **Ⓑ**

Labs and Diagnostic Studies:

Admission: STAT: electrolytes, blood urea nitrogen (BUN), glucose, CBC, cardiac enzymes, B-type natriuretic peptide (BNP), liver function tests; urinalysis; portable CXR; ECG, TSH

AM Labs: electrolytes, BUN, creatinine, glucose

Please obtain copy of prior echo report from Dr. Jones' office in the morning

Electrolytes and renal function are checked as a baseline at admission and checked daily during hospitalization. **C**

CBC should be checked at admission because anemia may contribute to HF. **C**

BNP should be checked if the diagnosis of HF as the cause of a patient's acute presentation is not clear. **A**

BNP tends to be less elevated in patients in HF with preserved EF (diastolic dysfunction) than those with low EF. BNP is lower in obese patients.

Cardiac ischemia, either acute or chronic, may lead to CHF. An ECG should be done for all patients presenting with acute symptoms, and cardiac enzymes performed if the ECG or history suggests acute ischemia. **C**

A CXR should be done for all patients presenting with CHF, both to support the diagnosis if Kerley B lines, bilateral effusions, or pulmonary edema are present *and* to rule out other causes of dyspnea, such as pneumonia. **C**

If this is the patient's first episode of CHF, check glycohemoglobin and lipid panel because diabetes and hyperlipidemia are common comorbidities in CHF and may contribute to CHF through CAD. TSH should also be checked at initial presentation as hyper/hypothyroidism may contribute to HF. **C**

All patients with CHF should have an echocardiogram to evaluate EF and to ensure that valve dysfunction is not causing CHF. Segmental wall motion abnormalities may also suggest CAD as the cause of HF. A repeat echo is not necessary for all patients admitted with an acute exacerbation of HF;

however, the inpatient physician should first review the echo
and consider repeating if there has been a substantial decline
in clinical status or if the patient does not respond to initial
therapy. ◉

Discharge Planning:

Effective management of HF requires good patient education. Difficulty with adherence to prescribed medications
and diet commonly leads to CHF admissions.

All patients should review the importance of a low sodium diet with a nutritionist.

Patients should also be counseled about the importance of
adherence to medications. A mediset may be helpful for
patients who forget doses. Medications may also be "blister
packed" by some pharmacies to help the patient take the
right drugs at the right time.

Patients should weigh themselves daily after discharge and
should be given specific instructions on what to do if they
gain weight; for example, "If you gain more than 3 pounds,
take an extra dose of Lasix. If your weight is not lower the
next day, call Dr. Jones."

Chronic disease management programs have been shown
to reduce hospitalization while maintaining quality of life for
patients with HF. If your hospital or clinic has such a program, consider a referral for your patient.

Post-discharge follow-up should be arranged for 1–2 weeks
after discharge. The patient should be instructed to call,
e-mail, or come in sooner if his or her weight rises to a certain
threshold or if he or she notices increasing edema or dyspnea.

Special Considerations:

Inpatient cardiology consultation should be considered for
patients requiring ICU admission, those not responding to
initial therapy, and those with suspected cardiac ischemia.

References

Abraham WT, Adams KF, Fonarow GC, et al: In-hospital mortality in patients with acute decompensated heart failure requiring intravenous vasoactive medications. *J Am Coll Card* 46:57–64, 2005.

Hunt SA, Abraham WT, Chin MH, et al: ACC/AHA 2005 guideline update for the diagnosis and management of chronic heart failure in the adult. *Circulation* 112:154–235, 2005.

Maisel AS, Krishnaswamy P, Nowak RM, et al: The Breathing Not Properly Multinational Study Investigators: Rapid measurement of B-type natriuretic peptide in the emergency diagnosis of heart failure. *N Engl J Med* 347:161–167, 2002.

Mueller C, Scholer A, et al: Use of B-type natriuretic peptide in the evaluation and management of acute dyspnea. *N Engl J Med* 350:647–654, 2004.

Nohria A, et al: Evaluation and monitoring of patients with acute heart failure syndromes. *Am J Cardiol* 96(6S):32–40, 2005.

Sackner-Bernstein JD, Kowalski M, et al: Short-term risk of death after treatment with nesiritide for decompensated heart failure. *JAMA* 393:1900–1905, 2005.

Syncope

Syncope has many possible causes and requires a thorough evaluation; however, for most patients, this can be accomplished as an outpatient.

Patients with a clear cardiac cause of syncope, or those at high risk for cardiac syncope, should be admitted for timely evaluation.

Specific risk factors that suggest the need for admission include:

- The history, exam, or ECG suggest a cardiac cause (e.g., a history of CAD or CHF, associated chest pain, palpitations, or a family history of sudden death)
- Age > 70 years
- Lack of vasovagal prodromal symptoms, especially in patients with other risk factors
- Associated with exertion
- Multiple episodes in a short time

Admission should also be considered for patients with:

- Injury due to syncope
- Suspected neurologic cause of syncope (TIA or stroke)
- Severe volume depletion

A dmit to: Telemetry

Because most patients admitted with syncope are being evaluated for a cardiac cause, they should be monitored on telemetry.

D iagnosis: Syncope

C ondition: Guarded

Patients with syncope due to cardiac causes have a high 1-year mortality, although it is often due to their underlying disease(s) rather than to arrhythmia or syncope.

V ital Signs:

Telemetry routine

Vitals are typically checked more frequently in telemetry units (i.e., q 4 hours). If severe volume depletion is the suspected cause of syncope, consider initially checking vitals q 2–4 hours over the first 12–24 hours to monitor the progression of volume repletion. ●

Allergies: NKDA

Activity: Fall Risk, Up with Assistance Only

For the first 24 hours the patient should be assisted each time he or she is out of bed because of the risk of recurrent syncope/falls. Activity can be increased if there are no further problems.

Once patients with orthostatic hypotension are able to get up independently, they should always sit at the edge of the bed for several minutes prior to standing. This should be reinforced prior to discharge.

Nursing:

O_2 to maintain O_2 saturation > 92%
Daily weight

Diet: Regular

IVFluids: Heplock IV

IV access should be maintained for patients on telemetry to allow rapid treatment of any arrhythmia.

If the patient is volume depleted, isotonic fluid should be given until volume is replete. Otherwise, IV fluids are unnecessary.

Medications:

Heparin 5000 units SQ 8 hours
Docusate 250 mg PO bid prn (hold for loose stool)
Hold furosemide

Discontinue implicated medications if possible. Carefully review the outpatient medications for any that may have contributed to the syncopal episode, usually by causing orthostatic hypotension or volume depletion. Remember that syncope in the elderly is often multifactorial, and medications may contribute significantly. Medications commonly associated with syncope include:

- Antihypertensives
- Diuretics
- Antidepressants
- Antianginals
- Analgesics
- Central nervous system (CNS) depressants

Remember that patients on bedrest need deep venous thrombosis (DVT) prophylaxis and may need a bowel regimen because bedrest can lead to constipation.

There is no universal treatment for syncope, but once a specific etiology has been determined, specific therapies can be recommended. For example, a beta blocker is usually first-line therapy for patients with recurrent neurocardiogenic (vasovagal) syncope, whereas fludrocortisone may be prescribed for patients with severe orthostatic hypotension due to autonomic dysfunction.

Labs and Diagnostic Studies:

CBC, Chem 7, CK, CK-MB, troponin now and in 8 hours
ECG
Echocardiogram

An ECG should be performed in all patients presenting with syncope because abnormalities may make a diagnosis or increase the suspicion of a cardiac cause. **Ⓑ**

Other routine labs have not been shown to aid in the diagnostic evaluation of syncope. **Ⓑ**

The history and physical (H&P) should guide initial lab testing. For example, if the H&P suggests volume depletion, check a CBC and Chem 7. If the H&P suggests cardiac ischemia, check cardiac enzymes. If H&P suggests a seizure, consider checking blood sugar, chemistry panel, and liver function tests (LFTs).

Further diagnostic tests should also be guided by history and exam, initial studies, and suspected diagnoses. Studies commonly performed in the evaluation of syncope include:

Echocardiography: For patients with known or suspected cardiac disease or an abnormal cardiac exam. If there is an exertional element to the patient's syncope, echocardiography should be done to rule out obstructive valvular disease such as hypertrophic cardiomyopathy or aortic stenosis. Patients who are exposed to dangerous situations (i.e., high-risk occupations) should also undergo echocardiography. **Ⓑ**

Testing for ischemia: Should be considered for patients with exertional symptoms or suspected coronary disease. **Ⓑ**

Holter monitoring: Should be performed if arrhythmia-induced syncope is suspected because of a history of palpitations, known cardiac disease, or abnormal ECG. **Ⓑ**

Electrophysiologic studies: Patients with known structural heart disease and syncope that evades diagnosis after the previously mentioned work-up should be referred for consideration of an electrophysiologic (EP) study. In patients with known structural disease or an abnormal ECG, the diagnostic yield is 50%. **Ⓑ**

EP studies are less useful in patients with no heart disease (yield 10%). Given the risks of this invasive testing, it is not recommended for patients with normal hearts and ECGs. **Ⓑ**

Tilt-table testing: Consider when a diagnosis of neurocardiogenic syncope is suspected or if syncope remains unexplained after initial work-up. Specific recommendations for situations to consider tilt table include: **Ⓑ**

- Recurrent syncope, or a single episode in a high-risk patient, and no evidence of cardiovascular (CV) disease
- If a patient has evidence of structural CV disease but appropriate work-up does not reveal cause of syncope
- If a clear diagnosis of neurally mediated syncope will affect treatment plans
- For evaluation of exercise-associated syncope

Discharge Planning:

Some of the work-up can safely be done in the outpatient setting as soon as immediately life-threatening conditions have been ruled out.

Outpatient studies: Holter monitoring provides 24–48 hours of continuous cardiac monitoring while the patient performs his or her usual activities. Event monitors are worn for a longer time and are triggered by the patient with or following symptoms, recording the cardiac rhythm around that time. If your patient has syncopal episodes daily, order a Holter monitor. If symptoms only occur weekly, an event monitor is more likely to make the diagnosis.

Patient education: Discuss risk of driving or other high-risk activities with the patient, especially if the syncope is recurrent or occurs in unpredictable circumstances.

For patients with orthostatic hypotension, provide:

- Education about sitting at the edge of the bed prior to standing
- A prescription for fitted, thigh-high compression hose, which may improve venous return and decrease the risk of recurrent syncope

Special Considerations:

Specialty consultation may be helpful in managing selected patients with syncope:

- Cardiology consultation should be considered for suspected cardiac causes and unexplained syncope.
- Neurology consultation is indicated when the history or exam suggest cerebrovascular disease or seizure (which can be difficult to differentiate from syncope).
- Psychiatry consultation may be helpful in patients with unexplained syncope, especially those with recurrent episodes or multiple somatic complaints. Anxiety disorder, somatoform disorder, and other psychiatric diagnoses are not-infrequent causes of syncope.

References

ACP/PIER: Syncope. pier.acponline.org/physicians/diseases/d250/d250.html.

Linzer M, Yang EH, Estes NA III, et al: Diagnosing syncope. Part 1: Value of history, physical examination, and electrocardiography. Clinical Efficacy Assessment Project of the American College of Physicians. *Ann Intern Med* 126:989–996, 1997.

Linzer M, Yang EH, Estes NA III, et al: Diagnosing syncope. Part 2: Unexplained syncope. Clinical Efficacy Assessment Project of the American College of Physicians. *Ann Intern Med* 126:989–996, 1997.

Hypertensive Emergency

Hypertensive emergency is defined as an abrupt, marked increase in BP that causes end-organ damage such as pulmonary edema, hypertensive encephalopathy, myocardial ischemia, renal failure, retinal hemorrhage, or papilledema. There is no absolute BP measure that defines hypertensive emergency; patients with long-standing severe hypertension can typically tolerate much higher BP without symptoms than patients with the acute onset of severe hypertension.

Most patients with elevated BP are asymptomatic and without evidence of end-organ damage and can be managed as outpatients with oral medications and prompt follow-up.

Patients with symptoms and evidence of end-organ damage should be admitted to the ICU for very close monitoring, telemetry, and initial treatment with IV medications.

A dmit to: ICU

Most patients should be admitted to the ICU or CCU for both intensive monitoring and IV medications that cannot be given on a medical floor. At some hospitals, patients with hypertensive emergency without cardiac ischemia may be admitted to a step-down unit.

D iagnosis: Hypertensive Emergency

C ondition: Critical

Symptomatic severe hypertension can have life-threatening complications, including aortic dissection, MI, renal failure, and intracerebral hemorrhage.

V ital Signs:

ICU routine, plus continuous BP monitoring with arterial line

Patients treated with IV sodium nitroprusside are usually monitored with an arterial line to measure BP continuously.

Those responding to initial therapy with another drug may be managed with frequent manual BP checks every 30 minutes. Frequency of BP checks can be decreased as the patient improves.

Allergies: Hydrochlorothiazide (HCTZ)

Activity: Bedrest

Patients should stay in bed initially but can get up with assistance once they are responding to initial therapy and any change in mental status is improved.

Nursing:

Every 2 hour neurologic checks; I/O
Call for SBP > 190 mmHg, DBP > 110 mmHg, any neurologic change

Because severe hypertension often affects the CNS, frequent neurologic checks should be done.

A dramatic fall in UO with BP reduction may indicate the kidneys are now underperfused. Consider allowing the BP to rise slightly and rechecking serum creatinine.

The level of BP you would like to be called for depends on the patient's initial BP and response to therapy.

Diet: Low-Sodium Diet

Patients with altered mental status should not be allowed to eat so as to prevent aspiration.

Patients should be counseled by a dietitian on a low-sodium diet prior to discharge.

IV Fluids: Half Normal Saline (NS) to Keep Open (TKO)

IV fluids should be limited so as to limit sodium intake.

Medications:

Sodium nitroprusside IV infusion. Begin at 0.1 μg/kg/min, and titrate every 15 minutes to achieve mean arterial pressure

(MAP) of 120 mmHg within the first 2 hours of therapy. Maximum dose of 5 μg/kg/min

Although no trials have examined the ideal rate of BP lowering, experts recommend aiming for a 25% reduction in MAP within the first 3–4 hours of treatment. Use parenteral agents for faster onset of action.

Drug choice in hypertensive emergency is guided more by clinical experience and expert recommendations than trial data because very few comparative clinical trials have been performed.

Sodium nitroprusside is a widely used, potent arterial and venous vasodilator and is effective for most patients but usually requires invasive monitoring and must be shielded from light. The drug should be titrated every 15 minutes until the goal BP has been achieved. Sodium nitroprusside is contraindicated in pregnancy and should be avoided in patients with renal or hepatic dysfunction. Patients treated with this drug should be monitored closely for signs of toxicity, including nausea, vomiting, headache, tinnitus, seizures, muscle spasms, and delirium. An alternate drug should be substituted if these occur. ❸

Alternatives to sodium nitroprusside include:

- IV labetalol. Can be administered either as IV bolus every 10–15 minutes or as a continuous infusion. It is contraindicated in CHF, bradycardia, heart block (second degree or more), and reactive airway disease.
- Fenoldapam IV infusion. Fenoldapam is a dopamine antagonist. It can be used in renal insufficiency but can raise intraocular pressure, so it should not be used in patients with glaucoma.
- Nicardipine IV infusion. Nicardipine is a vasodilator.
- Hydralazine IV is used preferentially in eclampsia. Because it causes reflex tachycardia, it is contraindicated in

myocardial ischemia, increased intracranial pressure (ICP), and aortic dissection.

- Nitroglycerin IV infusion. It is the agent of choice if a patient has myocardial ischemia or pulmonary edema or after CABG.

Avoid diuretics or beta blockers unless the patient has myocardial ischemia/infarction, aortic dissection, or pulmonary edema.

Labs and Diagnostic Studies:

CBC with smear, M7, urinalysis, CK, troponin, chemstick, CXR, ECG
CT scan of the brain

Labs and diagnostic studies should assess for end-organ damage, including hemolytic anemia (CBC with smear), renal failure (Chem 7), proteinuria or hematuria (UA), myocardial ischemia (cardiac enzymes), and pulmonary edema (CXR). **B**

If neurologic symptoms or signs are present, a CT scan of the brain should be done as soon as the patient is stabilized to assess for hemorrhage and edema. **B**

Consider a urine toxicity screen because cocaine and methamphetamine use can lead to severe hypertension.

The most common cause of hypertensive emergency is essential hypertension in an untreated or poorly compliant patient. However, after the patient is stabilized, consider testing for secondary causes of hypertension, especially if the patient does not respond to initial treatment. **C**

Discharge Planning:

Once BP is controlled (usually within 24 hours), add an oral drug and titrate the IV drug to off. The goal is to reduce diastolic blood pressure (DBP) to 85 mmHg over the next 2–3 months. Good initial choices are oral labetalol or a short-acting calcium channel blocker. More than one agent may be needed, and compliance is ultimately likely to be better with once- or twice-daily medications.

The patient should receive predischarge instruction from a pharmacist if available (on new medications) and dietitian (on low-sodium diet), in addition to the physician and nurse.

Outpatient follow-up should be scheduled within 1 week to reassess BP, ensure no end-organ damage, and review and adjust medications.

Special Considerations:

If the patient has had a stroke or intracranial hemorrhage, consult a neurologist if available for assistance with management, including BP goals, which are likely to be much higher to maintain cerebral perfusion. Rapid control of BP should not be attempted in this situation.

If hypertensive emergency is complicated by aortic dissection, BP reduction should be even more aggressive, with a goal MAP of 70 mmHg.

References

Cherney D, Straus S: Management of patients with hypertensive urgencies and emergencies: A systematic review of the literature. *J Gen Intern Med* 17:937–945, 2002.

Elliot WJ: Clinical features and management of selected hypertensive emergencies. *J Clin Hypertens* 6:587–592, 2004.

Hall WD: Resistant hypertension, secondary hypertension, and hypertensive crises. *Cardiol Clin* 20(2):281–289, 2002.

Aortic Dissection

In aortic dissection, the intima tears, forming a false lumen in the media and compromising blood flow in side arteries.

Patients usually present with severe chest or back pain but may also have symptoms related to compromised blood flow: syncope or stroke, MI, or limb ischemia. The dissection may cause acute aortic insufficiency or rupture into the pericardium or externally, causing shock and rapid death. Aortic dissections are divided into proximal (those involving the aortic arch) and distal (those not involving the aortic arch). Proximal aortic dissection is *always* treated with emergent surgery because mortality is more than 20% at 24 hours. Distal aortic dissection is often initially treated medically. A cardiothoracic or vascular surgeon should participate in the care of all patients with aortic dissection.

A dmit to: ICU

All patients with acute aortic dissection not having emergent surgery require admission to an ICU for very careful monitoring and IV BP medication.

D iagnosis: Aortic Dissection

C ondition: Critical

The 30-day mortality for proximal aortic dissection is 24%; for distal dissection, it is 15%.

V ital Signs: ICU Routine with Continuous BP Monitoring

Because reducing BP is the cornerstone of medical therapy, BP needs to be monitored very carefully, usually with an arterial line.

A llergies: NKDA

A ctivity: Absolute Bedrest

Patients should be on strict bedrest, avoiding any stress or exertion, to minimize increases in BP and shear forces on the aorta that could extend the dissection.

N ursing:

Neuro check q 1 hour. Check pulses in the legs q 1 hour and call if change. Monitor I/O, and call for UO < 30 mL/h. Call for SBP > 120 mmHg, DBP > 80 mmHg, HR > 80 bpm
    The patient should be carefully monitored for evidence of progression of the dissection, including change in neurologic function, pulses, or decreasing UO, indicating involvement of renal arteries.

D iet: NPO

Because of the possible need for urgent surgery and the risk of clinical decompensation requiring intubation, patients should be NPO. A low-sodium diet may be started when it appears the patient has stabilized.

IV Fluids: Half NS at TKO

M edications:

Labetalol 5 mg IV now, then 1 mg/min continuous infusion.
    Titrate up to achieve SBP 95–110 mmHg over the first hour
Morphine sulfate 1–4 mg IV q 1 hour as needed for pain
    The key to treatment is reducing BP and shear forces on the aorta, which extend the dissection. The goal SBP is 100–110 mmHg; the goal MAP is < 70 mmHg. ● IV beta blockers should be administered to patients with suspected aortic dissection while the diagnosis is being established unless *absolutely* contraindicated. The initial dose of IV labetalol is 5–10 mg, depending on initial HR and BP, followed by a continuous infusion of 0.5–2 mg/min. An alternative to labetalol is a continuous infusion of esmolol. If goal BP is not

reached quickly with a beta blocker alone, sodium nitroprus-side should be added. Sodium nitroprusside is a potent arterial and venous vasodilator, which should be started at 0.3 μg/kg/min and titrated every 15 minutes until the goal BP has been achieved. Sodium nitroprusside is contraindicated in pregnancy and should be avoided in patients with renal or hepatic dysfunction. Patients treated with this drug should be monitored closely for signs of toxicity, including nausea, vomiting, headache, tinnitus, seizures, muscle spasms, and delirium.

Labs and Diagnostic Studies:

Labs: CBC with platelets, PT, PTT, Chem 7, LFTs, CK-MB, troponin, ECG, CXR on admission. Daily CBC, Chem 7

Diagnostic studies: CT scan with contrast of chest and abdomen, to assess extent of dissection

If the diagnosis of aortic dissection is suspected, an imag-ing study should be performed immediately in the ED. CXR shows a dilated thoracic aorta in about two-thirds of patients but is an insensitive and nonspecific finding. **Ⓑ**

CT with contrast, transesophageal echocardiography, and MRI are all reasonable first tests, with high sensitivity and specificity. Because of the rapid availability of CT, it is the most commonly used test in many institutions. **Ⓐ**

If the diagnosis is strongly suspected but the first test is negative, another imaging study should be done.

Admission labs seek evidence of end-organ damage from compromised blood flow and provide a baseline. A CBC and Chem 7 are the minimal labs that should be done daily. If there is any clinical evidence of progression of dissection, appropriate follow-up studies should be done (e.g., ECG, cardiac enzymes, LFTs, repeat CT).

Discharge Planning:

Patients can be discharged when surgery is not planned, they are pain free, and BP is strictly controlled on oral medications, with goal BP $< \frac{120}{80}$.

They should be educated on the absolute need to maintain tight control of BP and should receive education about new medications from a pharmacist. A dietitian should teach about a low-sodium diet as an adjunctive measure.

Post discharge follow-up should be arranged within 1 week to check BP, exam, and labs. Follow-up imaging is recommended 1 month after diagnosis and frequently thereafter.

Reference

Tsai TT, Nienaber CA, Eagle KA: Acute aortic syndromes. *Circulation* 112:3802–3813, 2005.

Adult Diabetic Ketoacidosis

Diabetic ketoacidosis (DKA) can occur either as an initial manifestation of diabetes or in a known diabetic with superimposed acute illness, such as infection, stroke, or acute myocardial infarction (MI), or medication noncompliance. Patients presenting with DKA must be carefully evaluated for precipitating illness, which may present atypically.

A dmit to: ICU

Most patients with DKA are initially managed in the ICU because of the need for frequent labs, telemetry, and close monitoring. Mild DKA may be managed on a general medicine floor if frequent monitoring and administration of appropriate insulin can be done.

D iagnosis: Adult DKA

C ondition: Serious

Condition may range from stable to critical.

Mild DKA is defined as glucose > 250 mg/dL, pH 7.25–7.30, serum bicarbonate 15–18 mEq/L with anion gap of > 10, and alert mental status. Patients with moderate DKA have lower pH (7–7.24), lower bicarbonate with higher anion gap, and possibly decreased mental status. Critically ill patients with severe DKA have pH < 7, bicarbonate < 10 mEq/L, and obtundation or coma. **⊙**

🅐 Recommendation based on consistent and good quality patient-oriented evidence. **🅑** Recommendation based on inconsistent or limited quality patient-oriented evidence. **⊙** Recommendation based on usual practice, consensus, opinion, disease-oriented evidence, or case series for studies of diagnosis, treatment, and prevention of screening.

Vital Signs:

Postural BP on admit. BP, pulse, respiration hourly × 6 hours, then q 2 hours × 6 hours, then q 4 hours. Temperature q 4 hours

Patients with DKA are volume depleted at presentation. Postural vital signs can help guide fluid resuscitation. When postural hypotension and tachycardia resolve, IV fluids should be switched from isotonic to half normal. Tachypnea is a common response to acidosis but could also signal pulmonary infection, heart failure, or thromboembolism.

Allergies: Lovastatin

Activity: Bedrest × 24 Hours, then Up Ad Lib

Patients are initially at high risk of falls because of orthostasis and alterations in mental status. Ambulation should be encouraged when volume status is stabilized.

Nursing:

Strict inputs and outputs (I/O), capillary blood glucose (CBG) q 1 hour × 6 hours, then per insulin infusion protocol. Daily weights

Fluid management is essential for patient improvement. The patient should have two IV lines to allow for volume repletion and the administration of other medications, including an insulin infusion.

CBG is followed hourly for at least the first 6 hours of treatment, by which time the blood glucose is usually less than 300 mg/dL and ketoacidosis is resolving. At that point, CBG measurements may be made less frequently, guided by an institution's insulin infusion protocol.

Daily weights should be performed to assess volume status, and patients will receive large amounts of IV fluid. ©

> ## D iet: NPO Until Fully Alert, then Clear Liquids. As Tolerated, Advance to American Diabetic Association (ADA) Diet

Most patients are nauseous at presentation but may assist with rehydration by PO intake of fluids. Oral fluids should not be given to any patient with decreased level of consciousness because of the risk of aspiration.

IV Fluids:

#1: 1000 mL normal saline (NS) at 1000 mL/h
#2: 1000 mL NS with 20 mEq KCl at 500 mL/h
#3: 1000 mL NS with 20 mEq KCl at 250 mL/h
#4: 1000 mL $\frac{1}{2}$ NS with 20 mEq KCl at 250 mL/h
When blood glucose is < 250 mg/dL, switch to D5 $\frac{1}{2}$ NS with 20 mEq KCl per liter at 250 mL/h

Because DKA causes osmotic diuresis and vomiting, patients present with intravascular volume depletion and a free water deficit. Typical free water deficit in DKA is 6 L.

Initially, isotonic fluid is given to correct intravascular volume depletion, guided by the physical exam and urine output (UO). When intravascular volume is restored (based on assessment of jugular venous pressure, vital signs including orthostatics, and increasing UO), IV fluid (IVF) is changed to $\frac{1}{2}$ NS plus 20 mEq KCl.

This regimen provides 4–5 L of fluid within the first 8 hours of therapy. This should be sufficient to maintain urine output above 30 mL/h. ⊙

Pediatric and adolescent patients are at risk for cerebral edema with overly aggressive fluid replacement. Therefore, pediatric guidelines recommend less aggressive fluid resuscitation, not to exceed 50 mL/kg over the first 4 hours of treatment, and replacement of the fluid deficit evenly over 48 hours. ⊙

In general, hyperglycemia will improve before the ketoacidosis resolves and patients will need glucose added to the IV fluid once the sugar is below 250–300 mg/dL as protection from hypoglycemia as insulin is continued. **C**

Although serum potassium is often elevated at presentation, the correction of acidosis will drive potassium intracellularly and result in hypokalemia. Potassium should be added to IVF once UO is assured, and serum potassium is *normal*, before the patient becomes hypokalemic. For potassium > 5 mg/dL, or poor UO, no potassium is added to IV fluids. If potassium is 4–5 mg/dL, add 20 mEq/L; if potassium is 3–4 mg/dL, add 40 mEq/L. **B**

Acidosis also causes phosphate to shift out of cells, leading to initially high serum phosphate levels, but osmotic diuresis causes net negative phosphate balance. Phosphate supplementation in the form of KPO_4 added to IV fluids (instead of KCl) should be given if serum phosphate is < 1.0 mg/dL. **B**

Sodium bicarbonate is added to IV fluids *only* in cases of significant arrhythmias or severe acidosis (pH < 7.0) because IV bicarbonate can paradoxically worsen central nervous system (CNS) acidosis. **B**

Medications:

Regular insulin: 12 units IV bolus then insulin drip at initial rate of 6 units/h. Check CBG hourly

Insulin rapidly reduces serum glucose and causes potassium and water to shift intracellularly. Therefore, insulin should not be administered until potassium is > 3 mg/dL and hypotensive shock has been corrected. **C**

IV insulin accompanied by frequent blood sugar assessment is the treatment of choice for most patients with DKA. An insulin infusion is a safe and effective means of rapidly controlling hyperglycemia and correcting acidosis. The initial insulin bolus is 0.1–0.2 units per kg of body weight, followed by 0.1 units/kg/h. When blood glucose is less than 250 mg/dL, insulin infusion rate is decreased to 0.05 units/kg/h and adjusted thereafter according to a standard insulin infusion protocol.

Hourly subcutaneous injections of insulin lispro have recently been shown in one study to be as effective as an IV regular insulin infusion and may permit the patient with mild DKA to be managed on a regular nursing floor in some hospitals. ❸

Once the acidosis is resolved and the patient is able to eat, long-acting insulin (glargine or NPH) should be administered subcutaneously *before* the insulin drip is discontinued to prevent the re-development of ketoacidosis. The patient's usual rapid or short-acting mealtime insulin is also restarted when able to eat. ❸

Treatment of precipitating infection or condition is disease specific.

Labs and Diagnostic Studies:

Complete blood count (CBC), Chem 7, Ca, Mg, phosphate (Phos), liver function tests (LFTs), serum ketones, arterial blood gases (ABGs), urinalysis (UA), ECG, chest x-ray (CXR) on admit. Chem 7, Phos q 4 hours × 24 hours. Serum ketones q 12 hours × 3

In DKA, initial studies should establish the severity of acidosis, volume depletion, and electrolyte losses *and* establish the inciting cause of DKA. Infections such as pneumonia, urinary tract infection (UTI), and soft tissue infections may present atypically in diabetes, and cardiac ischemia may be silent, so initial UA, cultures, CXR, and ECG should be checked in all patients presenting with DKA. ❸

Other studies should be dictated by findings on thorough physical exam and initial lab.

CBG should be monitored hourly at first so that insulin can be adjusted.

Discharge Planning:

Patients should be able to eat and self-administer insulin and other medication prior to discharge.

Patients should also be instructed in how to manage diabetes on days they are ill ("sick days") to avoid future episodes of DKA. Teaching should specifically cover when to contact the health care provider early in illness and the need to continue insulin, along with an easily digestible liquid diet containing carbohydrates and sodium, even when sick.

References

American Diabetes Association guidelines for hyperglycemic crises in diabetes. *Diabetes Care* 27:S94–102, 2004.

Umpierrez GE, Kitabch AE: Diabetic ketoacidosis: Risk factors and management strategies. *Treat Endocrinol* 2(2): 95–108, 2003.

Umpierrez GE, Latif K, Stoever J, et al. Efficacy of subcutaneous insulin lispro versus intravenous regular insulin for the treatment of patients with diabetic ketoacidosis. *Am J Med* 117: 291–296, 2004.

Hyperosmolar Hyperglycemic State (Hyperosmolar Nonketotic Coma)

Hyperosmolar hyperglycemic state (HHS), previously called "hyperosmolar nonketotic coma," is a diabetic emergency precipitated by acute infection or other severe illness in a patient with type 2 diabetes. It is characterized by serum glucose > 600 mg/dL but, unlike DKA, no ketoacid production and normal anion gap (unless there is concurrent lactic acidosis due to hypoperfusion).

At presentation, patients are typically stuporous or comatose and profoundly volume depleted. Acute infection, cardiovascular or cerebrovascular disease, and drugs are the usual precipitating factors, but any acute illness in a type 2 diabetic may lead to HHS. About 20% of patients presenting with HHS have not been previously diagnosed with diabetes.

These orders are for a 79-year-old man with type 2 diabetes and 6 days of nausea and vomiting.

A dmit to: ICU

Most HHS patients require admission to the ICU, either for obtundation, severe volume depletion, or both. Occasionally patients are stable enough to go to a closely monitored floor bed.

D iagnosis: HHS (Hyperosmolar Nonketotic Coma)

C ondition: Critical

HHS is a life-threatening diagnosis. Mortality is high (~15%).

V ital Signs:

BP, pulse, respiration hourly × 6 hours, then q 2 hours × 6 hours, then q 4 hours. Temperature q 4 hours
Call physician for:
BP < 90 mmHg
Pulse >120 bpm
Temp > 39°C
RR > 30 breaths/min, urine output (UOP) < 240 mL/8 hours, any change in neurologic status

Patients will be volume depleted at presentation and will receive rapid IVF. Frequent vital signs are necessary to monitor response to fluids.

Neurologic checks every 1–2 hours are done because obtundation and coma are common in patients with HHS.

A llergies: Glyburide

A ctivity: Bedrest, Until Mental Status Improves, then Up with Fall Precautions

Patients with HHS usually have altered mental status on admit and are at risk for falls.

N ursing:

Strict I/O
Check CBG hourly, maintain 2 IVs
Daily weights

IV fluid is essential for patient improvement. The patient should have two IV lines to allow for proper rehydration and the administration of other medications and insulin infusions.

D iet: NPO Until Alert, then Clear Liquids as Tolerated, Advance to ADA 1500 kCal Diabetic Diet

Aspiration risk is high at presentation. Once mental status improves, observe the patient swallowing a sip of water prior to initiating a liquid diet—if any coughing occurs, consider a formal swallow evaluation before the patient is allowed to eat.

IV Fluids: NS Plus 20 mEq KCl per Liter at 1000 mL/h for 2 Hours, then Call MD to Reassess

The typical patient with HHS has lost 9 L of body water and is extremely volume depleted at admission. The first liter of fluid should be NS for all patients with HHS. For patients with hypovolemic shock, isotonic fluid should be continued until the patient is intravascularly volume replete, as judged by improvement in vital signs. Then the IVF should be switched to $\frac{1}{2}$ NS, to begin to replete free water. ◉

For patients with milder hypovolemia, IVF is determined by the corrected serum sodium (determined by adding 1.6 mEq to the measured serum sodium for every 100 mg the serum glucose is above 100 mg/dL). If the corrected serum sodium is elevated at presentation, the initial fluid should be $\frac{1}{2}$ NS. If normal or low, the initial IVF should be NS. Again, fluid should be switched to $\frac{1}{2}$ NS when volume replete. ◉

HHS causes marked potassium losses due to osmotic diuresis, and KCl should be added to IVF as long as the initial serum potassium < 5.3 mg/dL. ◉

When serum glucose < 300 mg/dL, IVF should be changed to D5 $\frac{1}{2}$ NS with 20 mEq KCl.

In general, hyperglycemia will improve before the hyperosmolar state. Patients will need glucose added to the IV fluid once the sugar is < 300 mg/dL. ◉

M edications:

AFTER serum potassium is back, if serum K > 3.0 mg/dL, give regular insulin: 10 units IV bolus then start insulin drip at 0.1 units/kg/h
KCl 20 mEq IV (in addition to KCl in IVF) prn serum K < 3.6 mg/dL

An IV insulin drip, accompanied by frequent blood sugar assessment is the treatment of choice. Blood sugar should be checked hourly, and when < 300 mg/dL, the insulin drip rate should be decreased to 0.05 units/kg/h and further adjusted per hospital protocol.

Once the hyperosmolarity is resolved and the patient is eating, long-acting insulin (glargine or NPH) should be administered subcutaneously before the insulin drip is stopped. Prandial insulin and correction dose rapid-acting insulin are also usually prescribed; *see* Diabetes Management, pp 275–280 for details.

Ongoing repletion of potassium will be needed. **B**

Treatment of precipitating infection or condition is disease specific.

Labs and Diagnostic Studies:

Admit labs/studies: CBC with differential, Chem 7, Ca, Mg, Phos, LFTs, CK, MB, troponin, ECG, UA and culture, blood cultures × 2, CXR, serum osmolarity

Follow-up labs: CBC qd, Chem 7, Ca, Mg, Phos q 6 hours × 24 hours. Serum osmolarity q 12 hours first day, then qd × 3 days

Admission labs establish the severity of hyperglycemia and electrolyte derangement and investigate the precipitating cause of HHS.

Osmolarity > 320 nmol/L is the main cause of depressed mental status in HHS. If mental status remains depressed after serum osmolarity has been corrected, other explanations of diminished mental status (e.g., meningitis/intracranial hemorrhage or infection) should be excluded. **C**

Discharge Planning:

Patients should be ambulating, able to keep up with nutritional support and afebrile, and able to self-administer insulin and other medication prior to discharge.

Social work should assess whether home support is adequate for these patients whose illness has typically progressed for days prior to admission.

Nutrition consultation may also be useful for diabetic diet review.

References

American Diabetes Association guidelines for hyperglycemic crises in diabetes. *Diabetes Care* 27:S94–102, 2004.

Gaglia JL, Wyckoff J, Abrahamson MJ: Acute hyperglycemic crisis in the elderly. *Med Clin North Am* 88:1063–1084, xii, 2004.

Umpierrez GE, Kitabchi AE: Diabetic ketoacidosis: Risk factors management strategies. *Treat Endocrinol* 2(2):95–108, 2003.

3

Upper Gastrointestinal Bleed

Upper gastrointestinal (GI) bleed (UGIB) is defined as originating in the esophagus, stomach, or duodenum. Patients may present with emesis of blood or "coffeeground" material, melena (black or maroon, "tarry" stool), or symptoms of anemia or volume depletion.

Gastroenterology should be consulted for upper endoscopy, which should be done within 24 hours for most patients, to reduce the risk of rebleeding for high-risk patients and reduce resource use for high- and low-risk patients. **Ⓑ**

Endoscopic findings, along with clinical findings, can be used to stratify risk of rebleeding.

- Small, clean-based ulcers, nonbleeding Mallory-Weiss tears, esophagitis, and gastritis are low risk.
- Larger clean-based ulcers, ulcers with clots, bleeding Mallory-Weiss tear or arteriovenous malformation (AVM) successfully treated are moderate risk.
- Bleeding ulcers, visible vessels, and esophageal or gastric varices are high risk. **Ⓐ**

These orders are for an 81-year-old woman with coronary artery disease (CAD) and atrial fibrillation, on aspirin (ASA) and warfarin, admitted with melena and a hematocrit (HCT) of 21.

Ⓐdmit to: ICU

The initial triage decision to the floor or ICU is based on the amount of blood loss, whether bleeding is active, and patient comorbidities.

Ⓐ Recommendation based on consistent and good quality patient-oriented evidence. **Ⓑ** Recommendation based on inconsistent or limited quality patient-oriented evidence. **Ⓒ** Recommendation based on usual practice, consensus, opinion, disease-oriented evidence, or case series for studies of diagnosis, treatment, and prevention of screening.

Patients with hemodynamic instability (i.e., severe tachycardia or shock), and those with bright red blood in hematemesis or on nasogastric (NG) aspirate are at higher risk and should be admitted to the ICU. **Ⓑ**

Patients initially requiring > 2 units packed red blood cell transfusion or transfusion of multiple blood products should also be admitted to the ICU. **Ⓒ**

ICU admission should also be considered for patients with known ischemic heart disease, heart failure, valvular disease, renal failure, or cirrhosis and for those with potential for respiratory compromise (i.e., massive hematemesis, altered mental status, or difficulty tolerating large volume shifts).

D iagnosis: Upper GI Bleed

C ondition: Guarded

The mortality of UGIB is 6–8%. Low-risk patients with no evidence of active bleeding are stable, but higher-risk patients are guarded to critical, depending on the bleeding source and patient comorbidities.

V ital Signs:

Per ICU routine. Call for HR > 100 bpm, SBP < 100 mmHg

Vital signs (VS) should be checked on admission and at least hourly for patients admitted to the ICU. On the general medicine ward, VS should be checked at admission, every 2 hours × 2, and if stable, every 4 hours thereafter. Increase in HR can be an early sign of recurrent bleeding. Continuous ECG monitoring is necessary for any high-risk patient, including cardiac comorbidities, ECG changes, or chest pain.

Allergies: Trimethoprim-Sulfamethoxazole (TMP-SMX) Causes Rash

Activity: Bedrest, Advance as Tolerated

Nursing:

Place NG tube and lavage to clear
Maintain two 16G or larger IVs at all times
Strict inputs and outputs (I/Os)
Deep venous thrombosis (DVT) prophylaxis with TED stockings (TEDS) and sequential compression devices (SCDs)

NG aspirate can help establish both the site of bleeding and severity of the bleed. Bloody or "coffeeground" NG aspirate confirms breeding proximal to the ligament of Treitz.

Bilious fluid excludes an active upper GI bleeding source because bile indicates the pylorus is open and blood is not present.

There is no value in checking the Gastroccult on NG aspirate.

Bright blood on gastric aspirate indicates a active bleeding, typically requiring ICU admission and early upper endoscopy. ❸

Maintaining adequate IV access is crucial for patients with active GI bleeding. Remember that triple-lumen catheters and PICC lines, because they are long and fairly small bore, cannot deliver as much fluid as quickly as peripheral IVs. For an actively bleeding patient, if adequate IV access cannot be maintained, consider placing a large-bore introducer sheath (Cordis) for access. ❻

TED stockings and spontaneous compression devices can be used for venous thromboembolism (VTE) prophylaxis in patients who are not ambulatory. Pharmacologic VTE prophylaxis in patients with active GI bleeding has not been definitively studied.

☐iet: NPO Initially

Patients should be NPO until after upper endoscopy.

In low-risk lesions, diet can be resumed after initial endoscopy.

For high-risk lesions, consider keeping patients NPO for an additional 48 hours in case rebleeding occurs so that repeat endoscopy can be performed more rapidly. ●

☐Fluids: Normal Saline (NS) Wide Open for 2 Liters, then House Officer (HO) Will Reassess

Isotonic fluid should be given rapidly until the patient is hemodynamically stable, then the rate can be slowed down.

Many hospitals have a supply of O-negative blood to be used for a bleeding patient in dire need of emergent transfusion prior to availability of crossmatched blood. For patients with GI bleed presenting with shock, emergent transfusion should be considered.

☐edications:

Pantoprazole 80-mg IV bolus over 2 minutes followed by pantoprazole 8 mg/h drip for 72 hours
No **aspirin or nonsteroidal anti-inflammatory drugs (NSAIDs)**
For patients with suspected esophageal variceal bleed:

- Octreotide 50 µg bolus followed by 50 µg per hour infusion
- Ofloxacin 400 mg IV qd × 7 days, first dose before endoscopy or Norfloxacin 400 mg PO bid × 7 days
- Propranolol 10 mg PO tid, starting when patient is stable and able to tolerate oral intake

In some studies, proton pump inhibitors have been shown to decrease rate of rebleeding, median hospital stay, number of packed red cells transfused, and need for repeat endoscopy. IV pantoprazole should be continued for 72 hours if endoscopy shows high-risk features for rebleeding. If endoscopy shows a low-risk bleeding source, switch to oral pantoprazole 40 mg PO bid, when the patient is tolerating oral intake. **Ⓐ**

Additional therapy and early upper endoscopy are necessary for patients with suspected variceal hemorrhage, who are at high risk of rebleeding and death.

Octreotide decreases splanchnic blood flow and decreases bleeding from varices. It is as effective as sclerotherapy for acute management of variceal bleeding, but combined therapy is more effective than either alone. **Ⓐ**

Prophylactic antibiotics should be given in variceal bleeds to decrease the rate of infection (mainly SBP). Prophylactic antibiotics may also decrease the rebleeding rate. This benefit is primarily in patients with Child's Class B or C cirrhosis. **Ⓐ**

Nonselective beta blockers (propranolol or nadolol) reduce bleeding risk and may improve survival. The goal is to decrease heart rate by 25%. The initial dose should be adjusted based on HR and BP and should be withheld until the patient is stable. **Ⓐ**

ASA, NSAIDs, clopidogrel, and warfarin should all be stopped in patients with active GI bleeding. **Ⓒ**

▌Labs and Diagnostic Studies:

Admit: complete blood count (CBC) with platelets, prothrombin time (PT)/international normalized ratio (INR), partial thromboplastin time (PTT), Chem 7, liver function tests (LFTs), ECG

HCT q 2 hours × 6

Type and cross 4 units of packed red blood cells

Type and cross at least 2 units packed red blood cells, more for high-risk patients. For the actively bleeding patient, also order and transfuse fresh frozen plasma if INR

> 1.5 and platelets if platelets < 50,000/mm³, to assist in hemostasis. ©

The HCT threshold for transfusion depends on the patient's age and comorbidities and acuity and severity of bleeding.

The frequency of HCTs is determined by the suspected source of bleeding. For very high-risk patients, while awaiting endoscopy, HCTs as frequently as every 2 hours may be needed. For hemodynamically stable patients presenting with melena, initial HCT order may be every 6 hours. Remember that HCT is an insensitive indicator of acute blood loss because a patient who has lost 1 liter of blood in the last half hour will still have a normal HCT on the remaining blood. ©

Check ECG on admission—if changes are concerning for ischemia, check cardiac enzymes × 3 (and admit patient to ICU or telemetry). ©

Test patients diagnosed with peptic ulcer disease for *Helicobacter pylori,* either with serology or biopsy, and treat those with positive results to decrease the risk of recurrence. ❹

Discharge Planning:

Patients can usually be safely discharged if there is no evidence of rebleeding within 48–72 hours, particularly with low-risk lesions.

Follow-Up Criteria:

Patients should return immediately for recurrence of signs or symptoms.

If the patient had *H. pylori* checked or biopsies were done, outpatient follow-up appointment should be arranged to follow-up on outstanding results.

For patients who have undergone variceal banding, a follow-up procedure may need to be scheduled.

S pecial Considerations:

Surgical consultation should be considered for any high-risk patients, including those with hemodynamic instability or massive or recurrent bleeding. **C**

For patients with esophageal or gastric varices, balloon tamponade with a Sengstaken-Blakemore tube can be used to achieve short-term hemostasis. Patients must first be intubated for airway protection, and the tube should be removed as soon as possible because tissue necrosis is a major risk. **B**

References

Aljebreen AM: Nasogastric aspirate predicts high-risk endo-scopic lesions in patients with acute upper-GI bleeding. *Gastrointest Endosc* 59:172–178, 2004.

Das A, Wong RC: Prediction of outcome of acute gastroin-testinal hemorrhage: A review of risk score and prediction models. *Gastrointest Endosc* 60(1):85–93, 2004.

Hayes PC: Meta-analysis of value of propranolol in preven-tion of variceal hemorrhage. *Lancet* 336:153–156, 1990.

Howden CW, Hunt RH: Guidelines for the management of *Helicobacter pylori* infection. Ad Hoc Committee on Prac-tice Parameters for the American College of Gastroenter-ology. *Am J Gastroenterology* 93(12):2330–2338, 1998.

Lau JYW, Sung JJY, Lee KKC, et al: Effect of intravenous omeprazole on recurrent bleeding after endoscopic treatment of bleeding peptic ulcers. *N Engl J Med* 343(5):310–316, 2000.

Minocha A, Richards RJ: Sengsten-Blakemore tube for con-trol of massive bleeding from gastric varices in hiatal hernia. *J Clin Gastroenterol* 14(1):36–38, 1992.

Soares-Weiser K, Brezis M, Tur-Kaspa R, et al: Antibiotic prophylaxis for cirrhotic patients with gastrointestinal bleeding. *Cochrane Database Syst Rev* (2):CD002907, 2002.

Lower GI Bleed

Lower GI bleeding is from the jejunum, ileum, or colon. Patients presenting with bright blood per rectum (hematochezia) usually have a lower GI bleed (LGIB), but NG lavage should be done to exclude a brisk UGIB as the source (*see* Upper Gastrointestinal Bleed, pp 54–60). Melena may be the presenting symptom of a LGIB from the small intestine or right colon but usually indicates the bleeding is coming from the upper GI tract.

LGIB is most frequently caused by diverticulitis, AVMs, colonic neoplasms, and hemorrhoids. Ischemic and infectious colitis and inflammatory bowel may also present with bloody stool.

Admit to: Floor

Most episodes of LGIB will stop spontaneously and will not recur, so many patients can be admitted to the floor.

High-risk features in LGIB include:

- SBP < 115 mmHg
- Tachycardia
- Syncope
- A nontender abdomen
- Active bleeding during the initial 4 hours of evaluation
- Aspirin use
- Three or more comorbid medical conditions **B**

Patients with high-risk features, especially active major bleeding, hemodynamic compromise, and unstable medical problems, should be admitted to the ICU. **B**

Diagnosis: LGIB

Condition: Stable

Most lower GI bleeding is minor and self-limited. Hemodynamically stable patients without anemia may be considered stable. However, patients with active hematochezia, hemodynamic instability, or unstable medical problems should be "guarded" or "critical."

Vital Signs:

On admit, q 2 hours × 2, then q 4 hours if stable. Call for HR > 100 bpm, SBP < 100 mmHg

On the general medicine ward, VS should be checked at admission, every 2 hours × 2, and if stable, every 4 hours thereafter. VS should be checked at least hourly for patients admitted to the ICU. Increase in HR can be an early sign of recurrent bleeding. Continuous EGG monitoring is necessary for any high-risk patient, especially those with cardiac comorbidities, EGG changes, or chest pain.

Allergies: NKDA, No Aspirin or NSAIDs

Activity: Ad Lib with Fall Precautions

Hemodynamically unstable patients or patients with active bleeding should be placed on bedrest. Fall precautions are appropriate for this mostly elderly population.

Nursing:

Place NG tube, aspirate, and remove
Maintain two 16G or larger IVs at all times
Strict I/Os
DVT prophylaxis with TEDS and SCDs

A nonbloody NG aspirate ensures that hematochezia is not originating from a brisk UGIB, which would be managed very differently. (*See* Upper Gastrointestinal Bleed, pp 54–60.)

Maintaining adequate IV access is crucial to management of active GI bleeding. Remember that triple-lumen catheters and PICC lines, because they are long and fairly small bore, cannot deliver as much fluid as quickly as peripheral IVs. For a hemodynamically unstable, actively bleeding patient, if adequate IV access cannot be maintained, consider placing a large-bore introducer sheath (Cordis) for access. ◉

D iet: Clear Liquids, then NPO After Midnight

Most patients admitted for LGIB will be evaluated with colonoscopy.

IV Fluids: NS 250 mL/h for 4 Hours, then HO Will Reassess

The initial IV fluid (IVF) management for patients with LGIB is the same as UGIB. After rapid initial assessment of hemodynamics and volume status, isotonic fluid should be given if the patient is euvolemic, then maintenance fluids should be given. Isotonic fluids should be continued for the minority of patients with LGIB with ongoing bleeding.

Many hospitals have a supply of O-negative blood for emergent transfusion. For patients with LGIB presenting with shock, blood loss has been substantial and emergent transfusion should be considered.

M edications:

Bowel preparation: for colonoscopy: polyethylene glycol–based solution (e.g., GoLYTELY) 1 L q 30–45 minutes with a goal total of 4 L
No aspirin or NSAIDs

If the patient is unable to tolerate the bowel prep by mouth, an NG tube should be placed for administration. Inadequate prep is a common reason for delayed or suboptimal colonoscopy—communicate clearly with the nursing staff about the necessity of getting the prep done, via NG tube if necessary.

Labs and Diagnostic Studies:

Admit: CBC with platelets, PT/INR, PTT, Chem 7, LFTs, ECG
HCT q 6 hours × 4, then twice daily
Type and cross 2 units of packed red blood cells

Admission labs should assess the degree of prior blood loss and comorbid illness. Frequency of HCT depends on initial presentation and whether bleeding is still active. HCT monitoring may be indicated as frequently as every 2 hours for patients with active bleeding and abnormal VS. **ⓒ**

Remember that HCT is an insensitive indicator of acute blood loss, because a patient who has lost 1 liter of blood in the last half hour will still have a normal HCT on the blood that is left.

Colonoscopy after rapid preparation is the preferred initial diagnostic maneuver and is potentially therapeutic for LGIB. If a source of bleeding is identified, endoscopic therapy can be applied. **ⓑ**

Angiography can also be used for both diagnosis and therapy of active LGIB, usually after colonoscopy has not revealed or treated the cause. Diagnosis by angiography requires a bleeding rate of > 1 unit/h at the time of contrast injection. Because of the risk of renal failure with IV contrast, it is not a good option for patients with chronic renal insufficiency. **ⓑ**

Tagged red cell scans are more sensitive than angiography, detecting bleeding as slow as a unit every 3 or 4 hours, but are also less specific. **ⓑ**

No randomized controlled studies of angiography and tagged red cell scans have been definitive.

D ischarge Planning:

Patients can usually be discharged if there has been no rebleeding after a period of observation (24 hours for minor bleeding, 48–72 hours for major bleeding requiring transfusion). ◉

S pecial Considerations:

A gastroenterologist should be consulted at admission. Prompt colonoscopy should usually be the initial test.

A surgeon should be consulted for all patients admitted with persistent LGIB, with urgent consultation for those with massive bleeding. Intraoperative enteroscopy to localize a site of bleeding, followed by resection of the involved bowel, is an option for patients with persistent bleeding of unclear source. Surgical resection should be considered for patients with persistent lower GI bleeding if a bleeding site has been localized by colonoscopy, angiography, or tagged red cell scan. ◉

References

Elta GH: Urgent colonoscopy for acute lower-gastrointestinal bleeding. *Gastrointest Endosc* 59(3):402–408, 2004.

Jensen DM, Machicado GA, Jutabha R, et al: Urgent colonoscopy for diagnosis and treatment of severe diverticular hemorrhage. *N Engl J Med* 342(2):78–82, 2000.

Strate LL, Saltzman JR, Ookubu R, et al: Validation of a clinical prediction rule for severe lower GI bleeding. *Am J Gastroenterol* 100(8):1821–1827, 2005.

Velayos FS, Williamson A, Sousa KH, et al: Early predictors of severe lower gastrointestinal bleeding and adverse outcomes: a prospective study. *Clin Gastroenterol Hepatol* 2(6):485–490, 2004.

Zuccaro G: Management of adult patients with lower gastro-intestinal bleed. ACG Guidelines. *Am J Gastroenterol* 93:1202–1208, 1998.

Zuckerman GR, Prakosh C: Acute lower gastrointestinal bleed. Part II: Etiology, therapy, and outcomes. *Gastrointest Endosc* 49:228–238, 1999.

Complications of Cirrhosis

Cirrhosis itself does not usually necessitate hospitalization. Usually, complications of cirrhosis such as encephalopathy, ascites, spontaneous bacterial peritonitis, GI bleeding, or acute renal failure are the triggers for admission.

These orders are for a patient with cirrhosis due to alcohol and hepatitis C, presenting with ascites and edema, impairing activities of daily living (ADLs).

A dmit to: Floor

A patient's mental status is the key to triage to the medical ward or the ICU. Patients with stage III (gross confusion or somnolence with intact response to noxious stimuli) or stage IV (no response to noxious stimuli; coma) hepatic encephalopathy require closer observation that may only be available in the ICU.

D iagnosis: Complications of Cirrhosis

C ondition: Fair

Adjust as clinical condition warrants.

Vital Signs:

Temperature, BP, pulse, RR, oxygen saturation, and neurologic status check q 2 hours × 4, then q 4 hours until stable, and then advance per routine

Patients can rapidly decompensate with worsening encephalopathy or hypotension, especially in the setting of infection or GI bleeding.

Allergies: NKDA

Activity: Up to Commode with Assistance and Advance as Tolerated. Elevate Legs if Edema Present

Bedrest for the first 1–2 days of a hospitalization theoretically may help to mobilize extravascular fluid, especially in the lower extremities, by decreasing activation of the renin-angiotensin-aldosterone system, increasing glomerular filtration rate, and increasing sodium excretion. ⊙

Bedrest for longer periods of time is likely counterproductive, and patients should be encouraged to increase activity after lower-extremity edema has improved.

Nursing:

Daily weights
Strict I/Os
TEDS/SCDs bilaterally
Guaiac stools
Clinical Institute for Withdrawal from Alcohol (CIWA) protocol for patients at risk for alcohol withdrawal (*see* Alcohol Withdrawal, pp 220–225)
Number connection test (trailmaking) on admission

Daily weight and I/O ensure that diuresis is occurring.

The number connection or trailmaking test is a standardized method of assessing the degree of encephalopathy.

Patients are asked to connect the numbers 1–25, randomly scattered over a sheet. This should take less than 30 seconds if encephalopathy is not present and takes increasingly longer as encephalopathy worsens. ❸

Diet: High-Protein, High-Calorie, Low-Sodium (1500–2000 mg/day)

In the absence of severe encephalopathy, a high-protein, high-calorie diet is indicated because most patients with cirrhosis have impaired nutrition. ❸

Limiting sodium intake to < 2000 mg/day facilitates reduction in ascites and edema. ❹

In patients with serum Na < 130 mmol/L in the setting of ascites and/or edema, restrict fluid to ≤ 1 L/day. ❸

IV Fluids: None

Maintenance IVF are not necessary if the patient is able to eat and drink. The sodium load in IVF can precipitate worsening of ascites and/or edema.

Medications:

Spironolactone 50 mg PO qd
Furosemide 20 mg PO qd
MVI 1 tablet PO qd
Acetaminophen 325–650 mg PO q 6 hours prn pain or fever. Not to exceed 2 g/day total
No narcotics or anxiolytics, please

In patients with ascites and/or edema, initiate diuretics (e.g., spironolactone 50 mg PO qd and furosemide 20 mg PO qd). ❹

Titrate spironolactone and furosemide to effect, but use caution because of the risks of prerenal acute renal insufficiency and hyperkalemia. Recommended weight loss rates to help avoid prerenal acute renal insufficiency are 300–500 g/day in patients without edema and 800–1000 g/day in patients with peripheral edema. **C**

In patients with hepatic encephalopathy, give lactulose 20 g PO q 4–12 hours titrated to goal of four loose bowel movements per day. **B** For patients presenting with severe encephalopathy, give q 1 hour lactulose per NG tube. Lactulose 30-g retention enemas q 4 hours are another option for patients who are unable to take PO but are less effective than oral lactulose.

In patients with esophageal varices, give nadolol (a non-selective beta blocker) 10 mg PO tid and advance as tolerated to goal of decreasing baseline HR by 25% while maintaining HR > 55 bpm and SBP > 90 mmHg. **A**

In patients with prior history of spontaneous bacterial peritonitis, give ciprofloxacin 750 mg PO q week or norfloxacin 400 mg PO qd for spontaneous bacterial peritonitis prophylaxis. **A**

Use narcotics and anxiolytics with extreme caution because these can precipitate hepatic encephalopathy.

L abs and Diagnostic Studies:

Admission: CBC with platelets; Chem 7; LFTs; urinalysis (UA); posteroanterior (PA) and lateral chest x-ray (CXR); diagnostic paracentesis fluid will be sent for cell count, differential, and bacterial culture
Daily: CBC with platelets, Chem 7

INR is the best measure of liver synthetic function. Follow HCT for evidence of bleeding and creatinine/potassium for changes with diuretics.

Calculation of Child's class requires bilirubin, albumin, and INR. Calculation of Model for End Stage Liver Disease (MELD) score for prognostic information and transplant listing requires INR, bilirubin, and creatinine.

Diagnostic paracentesis should be performed on every cirrhotic patient with ascites admitted to the hospital, regardless of the reason for admission, because spontaneous bacterial peritonitis is often asymptomatic and is present in 10–30% of unselected cirrhotic patients at the time of admission. Send ascites for:

- Cell count and differential—Spontaneous bacterial peritonitis is present if there are > 250 polymorphonuclear cells (PMNs)/mL of ascites. **C**
- Gram stain, aerobic and anaerobic cultures—Yield of ascitic fluid cultures is increased if 10 mL of ascites is inoculated into the culture bottles at the bedside at the time of the paracentesis. **B** A single organism on Gram stain and/or culture is most consistent with spontaneous bacterial peritonitis and can guide antibiotic choice. Evidence for polymicrobial infection suggests primary peritonitis as from a ruptured viscus.
- Albumin—This allows for calculation of the serum-ascites albumin gradient (SAAG = serum albumin − ascites albumin in g/dL). A SAAG ≥ 1.1 g/dL suggests the ascites is secondary to portal hypertension, as in cirrhosis. A SAAG < 1.1 g/dL is consistent with other processes such as tuberculous peritonitis and peritoneal carcinomatosis. **B**
- Total protein—Some authorities place patients on continuous spontaneous bacterial peritonitis prophylaxis if ascitic total protein is < 1 g/dL, but this practice is controversial. **C**

If the etiology of cirrhosis has not been previously diagnosed, assess for viral hepatitis with hepatitis B and C serologies; autoimmune disease with antinuclear antibody (ANA), anti-mitochondrial antibody, and anti-smooth muscle antibody; hemochromatosis with transferrin saturation; alpha-1-antityrpsin deficiency with alpha-1-antitrypsin level; and Wilson's disease with ceruloplasmin.

D ischarge Planning:

Begin patient and family education on cirrhosis. Education should focus on dietary issues, toxin avoidance (including alcohol and excessive acetaminophen), and management of chronic complications of disease.

Request social work assistance with resources for substance abuse issues if this is a problem.

Arrange follow-up in primary care and hepatology/GI clinic. If the patient is not actively drinking and otherwise reasonably healthy, refer the patient for liver transplant evaluation. Early referral is usually preferred.

S pecial Considerations:

1. Large-volume symptomatic ascites: Therapeutic paracentesis should be considered in addition to the diagnostic paracentesis in patients with respiratory compromise or extreme discomfort from abdominal distension. In patients with large-volume ascites, randomized trials comparing large-volume paracentesis with maintenance doses of diuretics versus high-dose diuretics alone favor paracentesis with maintenance diuretics. **Ⓐ**

   If removing more than 5 L of ascitic fluid, give 6–10 g of albumin IV per liter of ascites removed to help prevent circulatory dysfunction and subsequent renal dysfunction after paracentesis. **Ⓑ**

2. Spontaneous bacterial peritonitis: Start empiric treatment with cefotaxime 2 g IV q 8 hours. **Ⓐ** Antibiotics should subsequently be tailored if a pathogen is isolated. If resistant *Escherichia coli* or *Klebsiella* is present in your community, consider imipenem or a fluoroquinolone as empiric therapy. Optimal duration of therapy is unclear. A 5-day course appears to be safe in patients with < 250 PMN/mm³ of ascites and negative ascitic cultures 48 hours after initiation of antibiotics. **Ⓐ**

Give albumin 1.5 g/kg IV once at the time of spontaneous bacterial peritonitis diagnosis and 1 g/kg IV 48 hours later to decrease the incidence of renal insufficiency and death. ❹

Give continuous prophylaxis with norfloxacin 400 mg PO qd (or ciprofloxacin 750 mg PO q week), even after discharge, in patients with prior history of spontaneous bacterial peritonitis or spontaneous bacterial peritonitis during this admission because recurrence of spontaneous bacterial peritonitis is as high as 70% at 1 year without prophylaxis. ❹

3. Hepatorenal syndrome: This is characterized by rising creatinine in the absence of other potential causes of renal disease. It persists despite appropriate volume expansion and discontinuation of diuretics. Urine sodium is < 10 mmol/L. Treatment consists of vasoconstrictor drugs and albumin 1 g/kg IV at diagnosis and 20–40 g IV daily thereafter for 5–20 days. ❸

Vasoconstrictor options include midodrine 7.5–12.5 mg PO q 8 hours in combination with octreotide 100–200 μg SQ q 8 hours to achieve goal of an increase in mean BP of ≥ 15 mmHg, ❸ norepinephrine 0.5–3 mg/h IV, ❸ or terlipressin 0.5–2.0 mg IV every 4–12 hours. ❸ Terlipressin is only available in clinical trials as of 2006.

4. Vaccinations: Consider hepatitis A and B vaccines in patients without prior history of hepatitis A or B infection or immunization. ❻

References

Angeli P, Volpin R, Gerunda G, et al: Reversal of type 1 hepatorenal syndrome with the administration of midodrine and octreotide. *Hepatology* 29(6):1690–1697, 1999.

Blei AT, Cordoba J: Hepatic encephalopathy: practice guidelines of the Practice Parameters Committee of the

American College of Gastroenterology. *Am J Gastroenterol* 96:1969–1976, 2001.

Ginès P, Cárdenas A, Arroyo V, Rodés J: Management of cirrhosis and ascites. *N Engl J Med* 350:1646–1654, 2004.

Rimola A, García-Tsao G, Navasa M, et al: Diagnosis, treatment, and prophylaxis of spontaneous bacterial peritonitis: A consensus document. *J Hepatology* 32:142–153, 2000.

Runyon BA: AASLD practice guideline: Management of adult patients with ascites due to cirrhosis. *Hepatology* 39:1–16, 2004.

Diverticulitis

Diverticulitis is a common source of abdominal pain in adult patients, caused by inflammation or perforation of colonic diverticula. If an abscess, fistula, peritonitis, or sepsis is present, diverticulitis is considered to be complicated.

These orders are for a patient admitted with uncomplicated diverticulitis who is unable to take oral fluids and medications.

Admit to: Floor

All patients with acute complicated diverticulitis should be admitted.

Stable patients with uncomplicated diverticulitis may be treated as outpatients if they are able to take oral antibiotics and liquids by mouth.

Elderly patients and those who are immunocompromised should usually be admitted because signs of more severe disease may be subtle in these populations.

Signs or symptoms of a surgical abdomen, such as peritonitis, ruptured abscess, or sepsis, require close monitoring in an ICU.

Diagnosis: Diverticulitis

Condition: Stable

Patients with mild, uncomplicated diverticulitis are stable. Those with complicated diverticulitis are guarded. Patients with evidence of peritonitis or sepsis syndrome are critically ill.

Vital Signs:

Routine

BP, pulse, RR, and temperature are measured every 8 hours.

VS should be taken more frequently in patients who are more ill (i.e., hypotension, evidence of shock).

Allergies: NKDA

Activity: As Tolerated Up to Chair with Bathroom Privileges

Activity depends on the condition of the patient.

Elderly patients treated with narcotics should be on fall precautions.

Nursing:

Guaiac all stools
Daily weights
I/Os

Rectal bleeding is rare but possible in acute diverticulitis. Daily weights or I/Os are used to monitor volume status in patients treated with IV fluids.

D iet: NPO, Advancing to Clear Liquids as Tolerated

NPO is recommended for moderate to severe acute diverticulitis. If symptoms improve after 2–4 days, the diet may be advanced.

In mild episodes, a clear liquid diet can be given. ☚

A high-fiber diet is generally recommended after the acute episode is resolved. Avoidance of nuts and seeds should not be recommended because there is no evidence to support the role of seeds in diverticulitis and patients' food choices would be unnecessarily restricted. ☚

IV Fluids: NS 250 mL/h for 1 Liter, then D5 $\frac{1}{2}$ NS at 125 mL/h

Volume depletion should be corrected with NS, then maintenance IVF prescribed.

M edications:

Metronidazole 500 mg IV q 6 hours
Cefotaxime 2 g IV q 8 hours
Meperidine IM/SC 50–150 mg q 3–4 hours

Patients admitted to the hospital for diverticulitis should be treated with IV antibiotics covering anaerobes (especially *Bacteroides fragilis*) and Gram-negative coliforms for 7–10 days.

Appropriate antibiotic regimens include:

- Metronidazole 500 mg IV q 6 hours + third-generation cephalosporin

- Metronidazole 500 mg IV q 6 hours + ciprofloxacin 400 mg IV q 12 hours
- Piperacillin/tazobactam 3.375 g IV q 6 hours
- Ampicillin/sulbactam 3 g IV q 6 hours

Some authorities recommend adding gentamicin 5–7 mg/kg IV once daily for patients with sepsis and no evidence of renal insufficiency. ◑

Pain medications are controversial in patients with acute abdominal pain because narcotics may mask signs of peritonitis. However, after the initial evaluation, it is appropriate to provide pain control. Meperidine may cause less colonic spasm than other narcotics but has a toxic metabolite that can build up and cause seizures. It should not be given in high doses, for prolonged periods, or in renal insufficiency. ◑

Labs and Diagnostic Studies:

CBC, electrolytes, LFTs, amylase/lipase, blood cultures to exclude sepsis, UA and urine culture
Send stool for *Clostridium difficile* if recent antibiotic use
Plain films of the abdomen (flat/upright) and CXR (PA/lateral)

A CBC will show leukocytosis or a left shift in about two-thirds of patients with diverticulitis. A normal white blood cell count does not exclude the diagnosis.

LFTs, amylase, lipase, and beta human chorionic gonadotropin (HCG) (in women of childbearing age) are performed to exclude other causes of acute abdominal pain and are usually normal in diverticulitis.

UA and urine culture are performed if enterovesical fistula is suspected as a complication of diverticulitis. Urine protein and nitrates may be present simply because of bladder irritation from nearby diverticulitis.

Plain films of the abdomen and CXR are most useful for excluding other causes of abdominal pain, such as obstruction. Plain films will usually demonstrate free air if free perforation of an inflamed diverticulum has occurred.

A CT scan of the abdomen can determine the extent of disease and presence of complications. There are no data to support routine use of CT in all patients admitted with acute diverticulitis. Patients with a high pretest probability of disease and no clinical evidence of complications do not need an immediate CT. ●

CT should be performed for patients with severe illness, atypical presentation or unclear diagnosis, failure to improve with initial therapy, or a palpable mass that might indicate an abscess needing drainage. ●

Ultrasound has also been shown to give an accurate diagnosis of acute colonic diverticulitis (thickened bowel wall and abscesses), although it is very operator dependent and not used often in the United States.

Discharge Planning:

Counsel the patient regarding a high-fiber, low-fat diet. A low-fat diet is presumed to be higher in fiber. A high-fat diet typically slows bowel motility. ●

After discharge, when the acute episode of diverticulitis has resolved, the entire colon should be assessed for malignancy and for inflammatory bowel disease (IBD) with either a sigmoidoscopy plus barium enema or colonoscopy. ●

Patients should return to the hospital for increasing abdominal pain, fever, or inability to tolerate oral intake.

Special Considerations:

A general surgeon should be consulted promptly for patients with diverticulitis complicated by peritonitis, abscess, or fistula and for those who are failing initial medical therapy. Many abscesses may be drained percutaneously with CT guidance.

A general surgeon should also be consulted for patients with recurrent diverticulitis, in whom surgical resection of involved colon may be considered after the resolution of the acute episode, to avoid recurrent (and possibly more severe) attacks. Many surgeons also consider surgical resection after resolution of the first episode of diverticulitis in immunosuppressed patients, who are at higher risk with recurrent disease.

Right-sided diverticulitis is more common in young patients and persons of Asian descent and is much more aggressive.

References

Buchanan G, Kenefick N, Cohen CR: Diverticulitis. *Best Pract Res Clin Gastroenterol* 16:635–647, 2002.

Ferzoco LB, Raptopoulos V, Silen W, et al: Acute diverticulitis. *N Engl J Med* 338:1521–1526, 1998.

Mizuki A, Nagata H, Tatemichi M, et al: The outpatient management of patients with acute mild-to-moderate colonic diverticulitis. *Ailment Pharmacol Ther* 21:889–897, 2005.

Stollmann NH, Raskin JB: Diagnosis and management of diverticular disease of the colon in adults. Ad Hoc Practice Parameters Committee of the American College of Gastroenterology. *Am J Gastroenterol* 94:3110–3121, 1999.

Stollman NH, Raskin JB: Diverticular disease of the colon. *Lancet* 363:631–639, 2004.

Wu J, Baker M: Recognizing and managing acute diverticulitis for the internist. *Cleve Clin J Med* 72:620–627, 2005.

Acute Pancreatitis

Acute pancreatitis is most commonly caused by alcohol and gallstones. In about three-fourths of patients, pancreatitis is mild, without evidence of local or systemic complications.

These patients typically improve quickly and are ready for discharge in days to 1 week.

Severe pancreatitis is defined by local complications such as necrosis, abscess, or pseudocyst or by systemic complications such as systemic inflammatory response syndrome (SIRS) or organ dysfunction. Patients with severe pancreatitis are likely to require a much longer hospitalization and are at higher risk of death.

Several prognostic indices have been developed for pancreatitis. The Ranson criteria are commonly used, but the full assessment cannot be completed until 48 hours after admission. Patients with > 3 Ranson criteria during the first 48 hours of hospitalization have a high likelihood of a severe clinical course.

Ranson's criteria include:

At admission:

- Age > 55 years
- White blood count (WBC) > 16,000/mm^3
- Glucose > 200 mg/dL
- Lactate dehydrogenase (LDH) > 350 IU/L
- Aspartate transaminase (AST) > 250 IU/L

At 48 hours:

- HCT drop > 10 points
- Calcium < 8 mg/dL
- Base deficit > 4
- Rise in blood urea nitrogen (BUN) > 5 mg/dL
- Fluid sequestration > 6 L
- PaO$_2$ < 60 mmHg

These orders are for a 42-year-old man with recent heavy alcohol use, epigastric pain, nausea, and vomiting.

Admit to: Floor

Patients with mild pancreatitis should be admitted to the floor with careful initial monitoring. Patients with severe pancreatitis and those at risk for rapid deterioration, including the elderly, those requiring ongoing fluid resuscitation, and those with multiple comorbid conditions, should be admitted to a step-down unit or ICU.

D iagnosis: Acute Pancreatitis

C ondition: Stable

Patients with mild pancreatitis have < 1% mortality and are considered stable. Patients with severe pancreatitis are at substantially higher risk of death and should be considered guarded or critical, depending on presentation.

V ital Signs:

Every 2 hours × 3, then q 4 hours

The frequency of VS depends on the severity of illness and intravascular volume depletion at presentation. Even patients with mild disease should have frequent VS for the first hours of hospitalization. A rising HR, falling BP, decreasing urine output (UO), or increasing oxygen requirement all may signal clinical deterioration due to third spacing of fluid. Patients with severe pancreatitis should have VS every 1–2 hours until stable.

A llergies: NKDA

A ctivity: Up with Assistance

Patients with mild pancreatitis can get out of bed but should be cautious because they are likely to be receiving IV narcotics. Patients with severe pancreatitis should initially be placed on bedrest.

N ursing:

**Accurate I/Os. Daily weight. Assess and treat pain q 2 hours.
Call for SBP < 100 mmHg, HR > 110 bpm, temperature >
38.5°C, increasing O_2 requirement, or UO < 30 mL/h,
averaged over 4 hours**

Adequate volume resuscitation is critical to the initial
management of pancreatitis. UO, HR, and BP assess adequacy of IVF, while falling O_2 saturation is a danger sign of either
volume overload or noncardiogenic pulmonary edema due
to SIRS.

Pain management is also critical for patients with pancreatitis, who present with often severe visceral pain.

Historically, most patients with pancreatitis had an NG
tube placed. However, there are no data to support the
need for routine NG suction; only patients with vomiting
due to pancreatitis-induced ileus should have an NG tube
placed. **Ⓒ**

D iet: NPO

Patients with pancreatitis typically have pain and nausea and
are initially NPO. However, as soon as they feel hungry, they
may attempt to eat a low-fat diet. **Ⓒ**

Historically, patients with severe pancreatitis who
were unable to eat after several days were given total parenteral nutrition (TPN) to "rest" the pancreas. More recent
studies have shown that the majority of pancreatitis patients
tolerate enteral feedings, via nasojejunal or even NG tube.
Those treated with enteral feeds also have a lower rate of
infectious complications than those treated with TPN.
Therefore, pancreatitis patients should preferentially be
fed enterally, and TPN should be considered only if enteral
feedings are not tolerated.

IV Fluids: NS at 250 mL/h for 3 Liters, then Call HO to Reassess

Patients with pancreatitis are often intravascularly volume depleted and become progressively more so as inflammatory fluid leaks into the peritoneal cavity. Hemoconcentration is associated with severe disease, and experts have suggested that aggressive support of intravascular volume may limit the severity of pancreatitis. IVF should be given rapidly to correct volume depletion, but because losses will be ongoing, careful clinical reassessment will be needed every few hours to guide fluid choice and rate. **C**

If UO falls, HR rises, or BP falls, the rate of isotonic fluid administration should be increased as long as pulmonary edema is not developing. **C**

Medications:

Morphine sulfate 1–4 mg IV q 2 hours as needed for pain

Most patients will require IV narcotics for pain control. If bolus doses every 2 hours are not sufficient, a patient-controlled analgesia (PCA) pump should be considered. **C**

Antibiotics should not be prescribed for patients with mild pancreatitis. **B**

Patients with necrosis of more than 30% of the pancreas (on CT or MRI) are at high risk of infection of the necrotic tissue, which is a major complication. Antibiotic prophylaxis in this group remains controversial, with only some studies showing benefit. There is concern that prophylactic antibiotics covering Gram-negative pathogens have led to a higher incidence of infections with Gram-positive and fungal pathogens. However, most experts continue to recommend antibiotic prophylaxis with imipenem or meropenem for patients at the highest risk: those with necrosis of more than 30% of the gland. **B**

Critically ill patients should be treated with IV ranitidine for prevention of stress gastritis. **Ⓐ**

Labs and Diagnostic Studies:

Admit labs: Amylase, lipase, CBC, Chem 7, calcium, LFTs, PT, PTT
Abdominal ultrasound to assess for biliary cause of pancreatitis
AM **lab: Fasting lipid panel, CBC, Chem 7, calcium**

Both amylase and lipase can be used to support a diagnosis of pancreatitis. Lipase has a longer half-life and is slightly more specific than amylase. **Ⓑ** Serial daily amylase and lipase levels are not helpful in managing pancreatitis and should not be ordered. **Ⓒ**

At admit, the CBC and Chem 7 may already show evidence of intravascular volume loss, with hemoconcentration and renal insufficiency. Hypocalcemia is a marker of disease severity in Ranson's criteria.

LFTs should be checked to evaluate for gallstone pancreatitis; transaminitis is common early in the course of a common duct stone, whereas jaundice and elevated alkaline phosphatase may be seen later.

All patients admitted with a first episode of pancreatitis should have a right upper quadrant (RUQ) ultrasound to evaluate for gallstones as the cause. **Ⓑ**

Fasting lipids should be checked once because hypertriglyceridemia can cause pancreatitis. **Ⓑ**

A CT scan is not necessary for every patient presenting with pancreatitis but should be done *if*:

- The cause of abdominal pain is not clear.
- The patient has clinical evidence of severe disease on presentation, to assess for necrosis or other complication. Even patients without necrosis on initial CT scan may develop necrosis 48–72 hours later, however. If this is a concern, the CT should be repeated.
- The patient is not improving clinically after 3–4 days. **Ⓒ**

If the patient has fever or evidence of SIRS (both of which may be due either to pancreatitis itself or to infection), blood cultures should be performed. **C**

Patients with evidence of necrosis on CT and fever or sepsis syndrome will require further diagnostic testing to rule out infection of the necrotic tissue, usually with CT-guided aspiration of necrosis.

Discharge Planning:

Patients with mild pancreatitis are usually able to eat in several days and may be discharged when tolerating an oral diet and taking oral pain medications. Patients with severe pancreatitis, with local or systemic complications, have a much longer length of stay, often weeks.

Patients with gallstone pancreatitis should be evaluated by a surgeon for cholecystectomy. Because the recurrence rate of gallstone pancreatitis is high, cholecystectomy is often done before discharge. **B**

Patients with alcoholic pancreatitis should be counseled on the risk of recurrence with alcohol intake. If a diagnosis of alcoholism is made, treatment options should be reviewed by the social worker and strongly supported by the physician team. **C**

Special Considerations:

If a patient with presumed gallstone pancreatitis has evidence of biliary obstruction (elevated bilirubin or alkaline phosphatase, dilated common bile duct), gastroenterology should be consulted promptly for consideration of endoscopic retrograde cholangiopancreatography (ERCP). **B**

Gastroenterology consultation is also recommended for patients with severe pancreatitis. **C**

A general surgeon should be consulted for all patients with gallstone pancreatitis, as described previously, and for those with local complications, including pseudocyst, abscess, and necrosis.

Patients with pancreatitis may have severe SIRS even in the absence of infection.

References

Nathens AB, Curtis JR, Beale RJ, et al: Management of the critically ill patient with severe acute pancreatitis. *Crit Care Med* 32:2524–2536, 2004.

Shankar S, Van Sonnenberg R, Silverman SG, et al: Imaging and percutaneous management of acute complicated pancreatitis. *Cardiovasc Intervent Radiol* 27:567–580, 2004.

UK Working Party on Acute Pancreatitis: UK guidelines for the management of acute pancreatitis. *Gut* 54:S3, 20051–20059.

Acute Hepatitis and Acute Liver Failure

The most common causes of acute hepatitis requiring hospitalization are:

- Viral, especially hepatitis A and B. Hepatitis C, D, E, and G, herpes viruses, and Epstein-Barr virus are rare causes.
- Alcohol
- Drugs and toxins

Acute liver failure is defined as encephalopathy and INR ≥ 1.5 with no preexisting cirrhosis and clinical illness < 26 weeks' duration. Acute liver failure may be idiopathic or can be caused by any of the causes of acute hepatitis, especially drugs and toxins.

A dmit to: ICU

Most patients with acute hepatitis can be evaluated and treated as outpatients. Admission to the hospital is indicated for patients with:

- Acetaminophen-induced hepatitis, who require specific, monitored therapy
- Inability to tolerate oral fluids
- Evidence of hepatic dysfunction (encephalopathy, prolonged INR)
- Renal dysfunction, which may indicate more severe liver disease or volume depletion

Patients with acute liver failure should be admitted to the ICU for very close monitoring, and a transplant center should be immediately consulted for assistance with management and possible transfer. **Ⓑ**

D iagnosis: Acute Hepatitis and Acute Liver Failure

C ondition: Guarded

Patients with hepatitis should be closely observed for evidence of clinical deterioration, which may occur rapidly with acute insults.

V ital Signs:

Routine
Call for temperature > 38.5°C, SBP < 100 mmHg, HR > 100 bpm, and any evidence of sedation or altered mental status
Hepatitis alone does not cause hemodynamic instability. Acute hepatic failure is associated with a hyperdynamic circulation and peripheral vasodilation leading to hypotension.

The development of encephalopathy indicates severe illness, and patients should be reassessed promptly.

A llergies: NKDA

A ctivity: As Tolerated

N ursing:

Guaiac stools
Chemsticks qid

Patients with significant liver disease may be at risk for bleeding (from Mallory-Weiss tears related to vomiting or varices related to portal hypertension or coagulopathy).

Patients with hepatitis may develop hypoglycemia secondary to impaired gluconeogenesis. Chemsticks should be followed and rechecked immediately for altered mental status.

D iet: NPO; Advance Diet as Tolerated

Most patients with acute hepatitis have significant nausea. Diet can be restarted when nausea and vomiting have improved.

Patients with acute alcoholic hepatitis are often malnourished and may benefit from enteral nutritional supplementation, either taken by mouth or by feeding tube. These patients usually tolerate protein supplementation well, without developing encephalopathy.

IV Fluids: NS 200 mL/h for 2 Liters, then D5 $\frac{1}{2}$ NS at 100 mL/h for Maintenance

Many patients with hepatitis are volume depleted because of anorexia, nausea, and vomiting. IVF may be stopped when oral intake improves.

Medications:

Metoclopramide (Reglan) 10 mg IV/PO q 4–6 hours prn
Lactulose 15 mL PO tid—increase to achieve 3–5 loose stools
    per day
Avoid sedatives and narcotics

There is no specific therapy for acute viral hepatitis. Nausea is managed symptomatically with IVF and antiemetics.

Lactulose is prescribed only if there is evidence of encephalopathy.

If hepatitis is caused by alcohol, calculate the discriminant function (4.6 × [PT-control] + total bilirubin). If this value is > 32, creatinine is < 2.3 mg/dL, and there is no pancreatitis, bleeding, or infection, then initiate steroid treatment of alcoholic hepatitis—prednisone 40 mg PO daily for 4 weeks. Short-term mortality is high (> 30%) for patients with discriminant function values > 32, and steroids reduce mortality. **Ⓐ**

If hepatitis is due to acetaminophen overdose, initiate therapy immediately with N-acetylcysteine (Mucomyst) 140 mg/kg PO × 1, then 70 mg/kg PO q 4 hours for at least 17 doses *and* until clinical improvement occurs and INR is less than 2. Early consultation with a transplant center is indicated for those with encephalopathy, elevated INR, renal insufficiency, or acidosis because mortality is high among these groups. **Ⓐ**

Drugs are a common cause of hepatitis and of acute liver failure. Review the medication list carefully, eliminating all nonessential medications and all drugs that can cause liver disease, at least until the etiology of the patient's illness is clear. Even therapeutic doses of acetaminophen can cause hepatitis and liver failure in alcoholics. **Ⓑ**

Sedatives and narcotics should be avoided in patients with acute hepatitis, especially those with altered mental status. These drugs can precipitate severe encephalopathy. An exception is the patient with alcoholic hepatitis and alcohol withdrawal, who should be treated with benzodiazepines. **B**

Labs and Diagnostic Studies:

Admit: CBC, Chem 7, LFTs, INR, Hepatitis A, B, and C serologies, ethanol level, acetaminophen level, long toxicology screen
Daily: CBC, Chem 7, LFTs, INR

Alcohol and hepatitis A and B viruses cause most symptomatic acute hepatitis. Viral and alcoholic hepatitis can also cause acute liver failure, but in the United States, acute liver failure is most commonly caused by acetaminophen and other drugs. Even therapeutic doses of acetaminophen can cause hepatotoxicity in alcoholics. A serum acetaminophen level and a toxicology screen should be checked in addition to a careful history for acetaminophen-containing medications. **C**

Rare causes of hepatitis and acute liver failure can be evaluated with serologic tests on admission for acute liver failure or if initial evaluation does not reveal a cause for less severe hepatitis: ANA and anti–smooth muscle and anti-liver kidney microsomal antibodies for autoimmune hepatitis, and serum ceruloplasmin level for Wilson's disease. **C**

Discharge Planning:

Patients should be ambulatory with improving LFTs and normal mental status and able to maintain adequate oral intake prior to discharge.

Follow-up is scheduled for 1–2 weeks.

Special Considerations:

Altered mental status, rising INR, and renal insufficiency are all "danger" signs in acute hepatitis. Consultation with a hepatologist is recommended in all such cases, and appropriate patients should be transferred to a transplant center. **B**

Specialty consults to consider:

- Gastroenterology if the cause of hepatitis is unclear
- Transplant hepatology, at another medical center if necessary, in cases of acute liver failure

References

McCullough AJ, O'Connor JF: Alcoholic liver disease: Proposed recommendations for the American College of Gastroenterology. *Am J Gastroenterol* 93:2022–2036, 1998.

O'Grady JG: Acute liver failure. *Postgrad Med* 81:148–154, 2005.

Polson J, Lee WM: AASLD position paper: The management of acute liver failure. *Hepatology* 41:1179–1197, 2005.

Pratt DS, Kaplan MM: Evaluation of abnormal liver enzyme results in asymptomatic patients. *N Engl J Med* 342:1266–1271, 2000.

Small Bowel Obstruction

Most small bowel obstructions (SBOs) are due to adhesions from prior abdominal surgery or incarcerated hernias. Less common causes include neoplasms, Crohn's disease, volvulus, intussusception, and gallstones.

Patients with partial SBO are often managed conservatively on the medicine floor, with surgery only if the obstruction progresses or does not resolve with 48–72 hours of watchful waiting and supportive care. ©

There have been few randomized studies of management of SBO; the majority of these recommendations come from expert advice or usual practice.

Admit to: Floor

All patients with acute SBO require admission to the hospital. Patients with complete SBO require urgent surgery, whereas initial management for partial SBO may be non-operative. A surgeon should participate in the management of all patients with SBO. ◉

Patients with SBO may present with severe volume depletion, electrolyte abnormalities, and alkalosis from protracted vomiting. Initial management of patients with hypotension or severe electrolyte or acid base disturbance should be in the ICU if surgery is not warranted immediately.

Diagnosis: SBO

Condition: Guarded

In historic series, mortality of all patients admitted with SBO is ~5%, rising to > 30% for patients with complete obstruction and strangulated bowel at presentation.

Vital Signs:

VS q 2 hours × 4, then q 4 hours. Orthostatics on admission

Frequent VS are warranted during the first hours of admission as volume depletion is corrected and clinical status observed closely. Orthostatic VS can help define the degree of volume depletion.

Allergies: NKDA

Activity: Bedrest

Patients with SBO are managed with NG tubes to suction, which limit mobility.

N ursing:

NG tube to low intermittent suction (LIS), Foley catheter, accurate I/Os, including NG output

Call for increasing pain, temperature > 38.5°C, and HR > 110 bpm, UO < 30 mL/h

An NG tube should be placed in all patients with SBO. NG suction removes gastric juices and may prevent further distention but does not decompress the air and fluid already in the small bowel. Longer, weighted tubes do not seem to be more effective than standard NG tubes. **B**

A Foley catheter is typically placed to accurately monitor UO and guide fluid resuscitation and because the patient's mobility is limited by the NG. **C**

The nursing staff should be instructed to call for fever, increasing pain, and worsening tachycardia, all of which may indicate strangulation of bowel, an indication for emergent surgery. **C**

Low UO indicates inadequate volume resuscitation.

D iet: NPO

Patients with SBO should not eat until the obstruction has resolved or they are recovering from surgery, whichever comes first.

IV Fluids: NS 250 mL/h for 4 Hours, then 150 mL/h

Initial volume resuscitation should be guided by HR, BP, jugular venous pressure, and UO. Isotonic fluid should be given rapidly (250–500 mL/h) until volume is repleted and then continued at a slower rate (100–200 mL/h). Patients with SBO require more than maintenance IVF, even after volume deficits are restored, because NG suction can lead to significant fluid losses. **C**

Medications:

Prochlorperazine 12.5–25 mg IV q 8 hours prn nausea
Ondansetron 4–8 mg IV q 8 hours prn nausea not relieved by prochlorperazine
Morphine sulfate PCA per protocol
Heparin 5000 units SQ q 8 hours

Nausea usually improves with NG suction, but many patients require antiemetics. Prokinetic agents such as metoclopramide (Reglan) are *contraindicated* in SBO, so the best choices are dopamine antagonists such as prochlorperazine. If these are ineffective, a 5HT receptor antagonist such as ondansetron may help, but this class is substantially more expensive than older drugs. ⦿

SBO causes significant pain, which will require narcotic analgesics for relief. Every 2- to 4-hour IV bolus dosing of morphine sulfate or hydromorphone (Dilaudid) will be effective for some patients. However, if a patient requires more frequent dosing of pain medications, a PCA may be a better choice. ⦿

The patient's pain level and analgesic requirement should be followed closely and the physician team called for increasing pain, which may be a sign of bowel strangulation, an indication for urgent surgery. ⦿

DVT prophylaxis is indicated for these patients who are on bedrest and are likely to require surgery.

Labs and Diagnostic Studies:

Abdominal flat plate, upright and PA CXR
Admit labs: Chem 7, Calcium, magnesium, Phos, serum lactate; repeat Chem 7 q 8 hours

The diagnosis of SBO often can be made based on plain films of the abdomen, which show dilated air- and fluid-filled loops of small bowel. If the patient has had symptoms for more than 1 day, the finding of air in the rectum makes complete SBO less likely. An upright CXR is used to rule out free intraperitoneal air due to rupture of small bowel. If the patient cannot sit upright, a left lateral decubitus film can be done instead. **C**

If the diagnosis of SBO is not clear after history, physical, and plain films, a CT scan of the abdomen should be performed. A CT shows dilated loops of bowel and often the "transition point" between dilated and nondilated bowel, which indicates the site of obstruction. A CT can also identify signs of strangulation and ischemia and alternate causes of abdominal pain and nausea. **B**

Laboratory tests are not helpful in the diagnosis of SBO, but serum electrolytes are followed closely to guide the aggressive fluid and electrolyte replacement that is often required. Patients with partial SBO and less severe volume depletion on admission may require electrolytes only once or twice per day. **C**

Elevated serum lactate is a sensitive but not a specific finding in patients with strangulated bowel. **B**

Discharge Planning:

More than half of patients with SBO will require surgery prior to discharge. Patients treated nonoperatively may be discharged when nausea and abdominal pain have resolved and they are tolerating an oral diet. Patients should be instructed to call or come back for nausea, abdominal pain, or fever.

Special Considerations:

A general surgeon should be consulted promptly for all patients with SBO, especially any patient with complete obstruction or suspected strangulation at presentation.

Patients with complete obstruction or strangulation require immediate surgery.

The clinical diagnosis of strangulation is difficult. Clues include pain that changes from crampy to constant, worsening pain, leukocytosis, elevated serum lactate, hyperkalemia, and metabolic acidosis. If strangulation is a consideration, call your surgery consultant!

Even patients with partial SBO may require surgery if obstruction has not improved with 48–72 hours of watchful waiting.

References

Delabrousse E, Lewin M, Sournac L, et al: CT of small bowel obstruction in adults. *Abdominal Imag* 28:257–266, 2003.

Frager D: Intestinal obstruction role of CT. *Gastroenterol Clin North Am* 31:777–799, 2002.

Quickel R, Hodin RA: Clinical manifestations and diagnosis of small bowel obstruction. In Rose BD (ed): UpToDate. Wellesley, MA, UpToDate, 2006: www.uptodateonline.com; accessed 6/15/06.

Inflammatory Bowel Disease

Patients with inflammatory bowel disease (IBD) (Crohn's disease or ulcerative colitis [UC]) may require admission for:

- Severe disease not responding to outpatient therapy
- Complications such as abscess formation or obstruction

Although Crohn's disease and UC are distinct entities with differences in chronic treatment, initial therapy for severe disease is very similar.

Common indications for admission of patients with IBD include: ◉

- High fever
- Evidence of obstruction, which may be due to active disease or adhesions from prior surgery
- Vomiting and dehydration
- Rebound tenderness
- Toxic megacolon
- Anemia requiring transfusion
- Intraabdominal abscess
- Fistulae (in Crohn's disease)
- Cachexia requiring enteral or parenteral nutrition

The following orders are for a patient with severe UC admitted with worsening diarrhea and abdominal pain.

A dmit to: Floor

Most patients with IBD can be managed on a medical/surgical floor. Rare patients with systemic signs of sepsis require ICU admission. ◉

D iagnosis: IBD

C ondition: Guarded

Patients admitted with severe IBD may be seriously ill and may require surgery during hospitalization. With current therapy, however, mortality has decreased substantially.

V ital Signs:

Every 8 hours, check orthostatic VS q AM

Orthostatic VS can assist in following volume status.

A llergies: NKDA

A ctivity: As Tolerated

N ursing:

I/O, please record all stools, daily weights

With effective therapy, the number of loose stools per day should decrease. Following this trend may confirm clinical improvement.

An NG tube should be placed if there is evidence of SBO or toxic megacolon.

D iet: NPO

Patients admitted with symptoms of obstruction, severe disease (either UC or Crohn's), and possible need for surgery should be NPO. Other patients may have a diet as tolerated, but many are unable to eat because of the severity of their disease. TPN has not been shown to induce remission or improve outcome in patients with severe IBD, but if a patient is already malnourished and will not be able to eat soon, TPN should be considered. ⊙

IV Fluids: D5NS at 250 mL/h × 2 Liters, then Call MD to Reassess

Patients admitted with IBD may be significantly volume depleted. Isotonic fluid should be administered at a fairly rapid rate until volume replete.

M edications:

Prednisone 30 mg IV q 12 hours

Metoclopramide 10 mg IV q 6 hours prn nausea

Hyoscyamine 0.125 mg sublingually q 6 hours prn abdominal cramping

Hydromorphone (Dilaudid) 1–2 mg IV q 4 hours prn severe pain

Heparin 5000 units SQ q 8 hours

The first-line therapy for severe IBD requiring hospitalization is corticosteroids, 60–80 mg/day in divided doses. **Ⓐ**

Symptomatic therapies include antiemetics and hyoscyamine or other anticholinergic drugs to reduce abdominal cramping.

In general, opiate pain medications should be avoided if possible because they can precipitate toxic megacolon and may mask an acute abdomen. However, for patients with severe pain (after evaluation to rule out toxic megacolon or a surgical cause), it is reasonable to treat with low-dose narcotics while paying careful attention to the abdominal exam and other clinical indicators. **Ⓒ**

Diphenoxylate/atropine (Lomotil) and loperamide (Imodium) should be avoided in severe IBD because they may precipitate toxic megacolon. **Ⓒ**

IV antibiotics with Gram-negative and anaerobe coverage should be started for patients with abscess, systemic toxicity manifested by fever and/or bandemia, peritonitis on exam, or toxic megacolon. Ciprofloxacin and metronidazole is one possible regimen. **Ⓒ**

Other medical therapies that may be initiated if the patient with severe disease fails to improve, in consultation with gastroenterology, include IV cyclosporine and infliximab. After response to therapy, a variety of oral medications may be instituted for outpatient treatment and prevention of relapse, including azathioprine, methotrexate, mesalamine, and infliximab.

Patients with IBD appear to be at increased risk for DVT, so prophylaxis should be prescribed even if not at strict bedrest. Enoxaparin should be prescribed for higher-risk patients not having active bleeding, such as those with a history of prior DVT. If a patient will be discharged with an indwelling catheter, consider low-dose warfarin 1 mg PO qd, which has not been studied in this population but has decreased line-related thrombosis in another high-risk population, breast cancer patients.

Labs and Diagnostic Studies:

Admit: CBC with differential, Chem 7, LFTs, prealbumin, vitamin C, zinc level

Plain films of the abdomen—flat plate and upright, and upright CXR

Stool culture, and *C. difficile* toxin assay

An elevated WBC, especially with bandemia, increases concern for toxic megacolon, abscess, localized peritonitis, or very severe disease.

Hypokalemia may contribute to the development of toxic megacolon, so electrolytes should be carefully replaced. ☻

Prealbumin, vitamin C, and zinc levels can help assess recent nutritional status.

Plain films of the abdomen should be performed on all patients with severe IBD admitted to the hospital to rule out obstruction, toxic megacolon, and free air. CT scan of the abdomen should be considered if there is evidence of perito-nitis, high fever, leukocytosis, or bandemia, to evaluate for abscess. ☻

Occasionally, worsening symptoms in IBD are due to concurrent infection, most often *C. difficile* (because many patients have been recently treated with antibiotics). ☻

Cytomegalovirus colitis is also a possibility in immuno-suppressed patients presenting with a severe exacerbation; however, it can only be diagnosed by colonic biopsy. This is usually reserved for previously immunosuppressed patients who are not responding to therapy. ☻

Discharge Planning:

Patients may be discharged when afebrile, tolerating PO intake, or with enteral or parenteral nutrition in place. This may take only 1 or 2 days of IV corticosteroids for moderately severe illness but may take weeks (and other medications) for more severe illness.

Close follow-up with a gastroenterologist is advisable.

As you prepare for discharge, keep in mind the side effects of any medications on which the patient will be go home:

- Steroids: All patients should take calcium 1500 mg/day and vitamin D 400 IU/day for osteoporosis prevention. Consider a DEXA scan for patients who have had substantial past steroid treatment. If osteoporosis is already present, a bisphosphonate should be started.
- Azathioprine and 6-MP: Patients with a genetic defect in production of thiopurine methyl transferase (TPMT) are at increased risk for bone marrow toxicity. In addition to the weekly CBC routinely recommended for the first month that a patient is on these drugs, genetic testing for abnormal TPMT may be done.
- Infliximab: Patients are at markedly increased risk for reactivation tuberculosis (TB) because TNF is partly responsible for the granulomas that keep latent TB "in check." A purified protein derivative (PPD) should be performed in all patients being treated with infliximab.

Special Considerations:

Gastroenterology consultation is appropriate for all patients with IBD who are sick enough to be admitted to the hospital.

Toxic megacolon is characterized by dilatation of the colon (> 6 cm) with evidence of systemic toxicity and may occur either in UC or Crohn's disease. It is an indication for surgical consultation, NG suction, very close monitoring (possibly in the ICU), discontinuation of all opiates and anticholinergics, and colonic resection if the clinical condition deteriorates or does not improve after several days of medical therapy.

Other indications for surgical consultation in IBD are:

- Peritonitis
- Intraabdominal abscess (which may be managed surgically or with percutaneous drains)
- Refractory disease
- Obstruction not responsive to medical therapy

References

Carter MJ, Lobo AJ, Travis SP: Guidelines for the management of inflammatory bowel disease in adults. *Gut* 53(Suppl 5):V1–16, 2004.

Hanauer SB, Sandborn W: Management of Crohn's disease in adults. *Am J Gastroenterol* 96:635–643, 2001.

Nikolaus S, Rutgerts P, Fedorak R, et al: Interferon beta-1a in ulcerative colitis: a placebo controlled, randomised, dose escalating study. *Gut* 52:1286–1290, 2003. Erratum in: *Gut* 52:1657, 2003.

Su C, Salzberg BA, Lewis JD, et al: Efficacy of anti-tumor necrosis factor therapy in patients with ulcerative colitis. *Am J Gastroenterol* 97:2577–2584, 2002.

Targan SR, Hanauer SB, van Deventer SJ, et al: A short-term study of chimeric monoclonal antibody cA2 to tumor necrosis factor alpha for Crohn's disease. Crohn's Disease cA2 Study Group. *N Engl J Med* 337:1029–1035, 1997.

Cholecystitis

Cholecystitis presents with RUQ pain, fever, and leukocytosis, usually in a patient with gallstones. Twelve percent of the population has gallstones, but most are asymptomatic. Passage of a stone through the cystic duct causes epigastric or RUQ pain, lasting minutes to a few hours. Pain lasting longer than 4 hours should suggest cholecystitis, especially if accompanied by fever.

Chronically ill patients can also develop cholecystitis without gallstones, which is called *acalculous cholecystitis* and has much higher morbidity and mortality.

A surgeon should be consulted to plan for and determine the timing of cholecystectomy performed in most patients.

These orders are for a 52-year-old woman admitted with 1 day of RUQ pain and fever, accompanied by nausea and vomiting.

A dmit to: Floor

Patients with cholecystitis are usually stable enough to be admitted to the floor. However, patients with cholecystitis may develop cholangitis (*see* Cholangitis, pp 106–110), gangrene, or perforation of the gallbladder, all of which are life threatening.

Patients with cholecystitis should have frequent abdominal exams to detect complications requiring emergent surgery.

D iagnosis: Cholecystitis

C ondition: Stable

Patients with evidence of complications (cholangitis, gangrene, perforation) are critically ill.

V ital Signs:

**VS on admission, then q 4 hours. Call for HR > 120 bpm,
SBP < 100 mmHg, RR > 28 breaths/minute, decreasing UO**
VS abnormalities can be an early sign of sepsis.

A llergies: NKDA

A ctivity: As Tolerated. Fall Precautions

Fall precautions are appropriate for patients treated with opiates.

If an NG tube is placed for relief of vomiting, the patient should be on bedrest.

N ursing:

Weight on admission, strict I/Os
Decreasing UO can be an early sign of sepsis.

D iet: NPO

NPO should be ordered initially, with advancement of diets to clear liquids and then to low fat as the patient clinically improves.

NPO past midnight is recommended on the day of cholecystectomy.

IV Fluids: NS at 250 mL/h, then Begin D5 $\frac{1}{2}$ NS at 125 mL/h

Patients who have been vomiting or have had symptoms for days may be quite volume depleted at presentation. Isotonic fluid should be given until volume is repleted, then switched to maintenance fluid.

Medications:

Ampicillin 2 g IV q 4 hours
Gentamicin 5 mg/kg IV q 24 hours
Morphine sulfate 1–5 mg IV q 1 hour prn pain

Cholecystitis is caused by inflammation of the gallbladder, with or without infection. There are no clear trial data supporting the use of a given antibiotic regimen, but patients with cholecystitis are treated to cover the usual pathogens: Gram-negative rods, including *E. coli, Klebsiella,* and *Enterobacter* species, and *Enterococcus*. Ampicillin and gentamicin is the traditional regimen for cholecystitis. Gentamicin should be avoided in patients with renal insufficiency, cirrhosis, or diabetes. ●

Other reasonable antibiotic regimens include a carbapenem, a fluoroquinolone, ampicillin-sulbactam, ticarcillin clavulanate, or piperacillin-tazobactam.

If sampling of bile is done (via urgent surgery, or cholecystostomy), the bile should be sent for culture to help direct antibiotic therapy. ●

Patients with cholecystitis usually require pain medications, often opiates. Ketorolac has been studied and found to be effective but should be avoided if the patient is volume depleted, has heart failure, or is on another nephrotoxic medication (i.e., gentamicin).

Labs and Diagnostic Studies:

**Admission: CBC with differential, LFTs, amylase, basic metabolic
    panel, and blood cultures × 2**
RUQ ultrasound
Daily CBC, LFTs
ECG

WBC is usually elevated, often with left shift. Mild LFT abnormalities may occur in cholecystitis, but significant increase in bilirubin or alkaline phosphatase should suggest biliary obstruction or cholangitis. Blood cultures are not usually positive but should be done.

The sensitivity of ultrasound in diagnosing acute cholecystitis is 88%, and the specificity is 80%. **Ⓐ**

A HIDA scan should be performed if the diagnosis of cholecystitis is uncertain after ultrasound because this scan has a higher sensitivity and specificity. **Ⓑ**

D ischarge Planning:

Hospital length of stay will depend on the severity of illness and the timing of cholecystectomy.

Most patients are ready for discharge on the day following laparoscopic cholecystectomy, but hospitalization will be longer if an open procedure is needed.

S pecial Considerations:

Patients with one episode of cholecystitis are at high risk for recurrence, with its attendant risk of complications. Therefore, all but very high-risk patients should have cholecystectomy. Once patients become symptomatic, they should undergo cholecystectomy on the next available operative day, **Ⓑ** which decreases hospital stay but does not decrease complication rate.

Patients with cholecystitis should usually have cholecystectomy performed within 72 hours. **Ⓑ**

Patients whose surgical risk is excessive may be managed with antibiotics for the first 1–2 days, with placement of a cholecystostomy tube for drainage of the gallbladder if unimproved. **Ⓒ**

References

Bellows CF, Berger DH, Crass RA, et al: Management of gallstones. *Am Fam Physician* 72:637–642, 2005.

Cirillo D, Wallace RB, Radabough RI, et al: Effect of estrogen therapy on gallbladder disease. *JAMA* 293:330–339, 2005.

Johansen EC, Madoff LC: Infections of the biliary system. In Mandell, Bennett, Dolan (eds): *Principles and Practice of Infectious Disease*, ed 6. Churchill Livingstone, 2005, pp 955–958.

Papi C, Catarci M, D'Ambrosio L, et al: Timing of cholecystectomy for acute calculous cholecystitis: a meta-analysis. *Am J Gastroenterol* 99:147–155, 2004.

Cholangitis

Cholangitis is caused by bacterial infection of the biliary tract, usually in the setting of obstruction. Prior manipulation of the biliary tree (papillotomy, stent placement, recent ERCP) increases risk.

Cholangitis should be considered in any patient who presents with symptoms of RUQ pain, fever, and jaundice. However, only 50–75% of patients have this classic triad.

The severity of illness ranges from mild to critical.

These orders are for a 61-year-old man with known pancreatic cancer, presenting with fever but otherwise stable VS, RUQ pain, and jaundice.

Admit to: Floor

Patients with cholangitis may be clinically stable to critically ill. They can be admitted to the floor with frequent VS if clinically stable but should be admitted to the ICU if there is evidence of sepsis.

A gastroenterology consult for consideration of ERCP should be obtained, urgently if there is evidence of sepsis.

A surgeon should also be consulted for patients with sepsis. ☻

D iagnosis: Cholangitis

C ondition: Serious

Patients with cholangitis are at risk of rapidly progressive infection.

V ital Signs:

VS on admit and q 2 hours overnight. Call for HR > 100 bpm, SBP < 110 mmHg, increased RR, or decreased UO

If a patient with cholangitis is admitted to the floor, close monitoring for evidence of sepsis is essential.

A llergies: Codeine

A ctivity: Bedrest Until Stable

Fall precautions would also be appropriate for opiate-treated patients.

N ursing:

Weight on admission, strict I/Os

D iet: NPO

When the patient is clinically improving, advance diet slowly, starting with clear liquids. Keep the patient NPO if urgent ERCP or surgery could be necessary. ☻

IV Fluids: NS 250 mL/h for 8 Hours, then Start D5 $\frac{1}{2}$ NS at 125 mL/h

IVF will be guided by a patient's presentation and exam. Patients who have had decreased oral intake for several days will require more aggressive isotonic fluid replacement, as will patients with sepsis.

Once the patient is volume replete and stable, maintenance fluids should be continued until the patient is able to eat normally.

Medications:

Ampicillin 2 g IV q 4 hours
Gentamicin 5 mg/kg IV q 24 hours
Morphine sulfate 1–5 mg IV q 1 hour prn pain

The usual pathogens in cholangitis are Gram-negative rods (*E. coli, Klebsiella, Enterobacter* species) and enterococcus. Initial empiric therapy should cover these organisms. Ampicillin plus gentamicin is the traditional regimen, with or without anaerobic coverage by metronidazole. Gentamicin should be avoided in patients with renal insufficiency, cirrhosis, or diabetes. **ⓑ**

Other reasonable antibiotic regimens include a carbapenem, a fluoroquinolone, ampicillin-sulbactam, ticarcillin clavulanate, or piperacillin-tazobactam.

Pain medication is usually necessary.

If the patient has sepsis, *see* Severe Sepsis and Septic Shock, pp 182–189 for further therapies.

Labs and Diagnostic Studies:

CBC with differential, LFTs, amylase, basic metabolic panel, PT, PTT, and blood cultures × 2 on admission
Daily CBC, Chem 7, LFTs
RUQ ultrasound
Anticipate ERCP in AM

Most patients with cholangitis have leukocytosis, and blood cultures are positive in 50%. LFTs are typically abnormal with a cholestatic pattern due to biliary obstruction, and amylase may be elevated, indicating an associated pancreatitis.

If sampling of bile is done (via ERCP), the bile should be sent for culture to help direct antibiotic therapy, as should any hardware or stents removed from the biliary tree.

RUQ ultrasound should be done at admission to detect biliary obstruction/dilatation, which support the diagnosis of cholangitis. **❸**

ERCP is both diagnostic and therapeutic because stones can be removed and obstruction relieved with stent or sphincterotomy. **❸**

Magnetic resonance cholangiopancreatography (MRCP) may be considered in patients for whom ERCP will be difficult or in whom an ERCP has been incomplete and who are not seriously ill. It has a high sensitivity (compared with the gold standard of ERCP), but therapeutic interventions cannot be made.

Discharge Planning:

Length of hospitalization and postdischarge needs will depend on the cause of cholangitis, as well as the severity of illness.

Patients with choledocholithiasis or cholelithiasis should have their gallbladder removed plus intraoperative common bile duct exploration, usually prior to discharge from the hospital.

Patients with cholangitis in the setting of obstruction previously treated with a biliary stent usually improve quickly after stent replacement, although recurrent episodes may occur.

Special Considerations:

ERCP should be performed urgently to relieve biliary obstruction in patients presenting with cholangitis and sepsis. ☉

If ERCP is unsuccessful, percutaneous drainage of the biliary system may be attempted by interventional radiology.

References

Barish MA, Yucel EK, Ferruci JT, et al: Current concepts: Magnetic resonance cholangiopancreatography. *N Engl J Med* 341:258–264, 1999.

Johansen EC, Madoff LC: Infections of the biliary system. In Mandell, Bennett, Dolan (eds): *Principles and Practice of Infectious Disease*, ed 6. Churchill Livingstone, 2005, pp 955–958.

Gastroparesis

Most gastroparesis is caused by longstanding diabetes, but it may also be idiopathic or caused by diseases of the autonomic nervous system.

Patients with severe chronic gastroparesis may require hospital admission for symptom management, treatment of volume depletion, and correction of electrolyte abnormalities.

These orders are for a 32-year-old man with type 1 diabetes who has been admitted four times in the last 5 months with severe nausea, vomiting, and volume depletion.

Admit to: Floor

Most patients with gastroparesis can be managed on the medical floor. Patients with diabetic gastroparesis, especially type 1 diabetics, require close monitoring of blood glucose and insulin management until the usual dietary intake is restored. Hyperglycemia worsens gastroparesis, and symptoms may not improve until blood sugar is brought under control. ❽

D iagnosis: Gastroparesis

C ondition: Stable

When admission is required, symptoms are refractory and volume depletion is often present. Patients with type 1 diabetes mellitus often present with concomitant diabetic ketoacidosis (DKA).

V ital Signs:

Routine. Check orthostatic VS on admission and once per shift × 3

Orthostatic VS can help guide volume resuscitation.

A llergies: NKDA

A ctivity: Out of Bed with Assistance

Most patients with severe gastroparesis requiring hospital admission are initially not well enough to ambulate independently. Orthostasis due to volume depletion must be corrected prior to safe ambulation. As symptoms improve, increased activity should be encouraged.

N ursing:

Finger-stick blood sugar checks per insulin drip protocol

Patients with type 1 diabetes mellitus are treated with an insulin drip or long-acting SQ insulin plus supplemental

hydration is often helpful to look for occult anemia that may not be apparent on admission. Women of childbearing age should receive a serum pregnancy test. ⊙

For patients with established gastroparesis, following serial gastric emptying studies is usually not necessary because clinical symptoms can be followed. ⊙

For patients with previously undiagnosed gastroparesis, a nuclear medicine gastric emptying study assist in the diagnosis. Other causes of similar symptoms may need to be evaluated, including upper endoscopy or upper GI series to rule out obstruction in the upper GI tract, abdominal plain films to rule out SBO, and urine toxicology screen for occult substance abuse. Once delayed gastric emptying is identified, an investigation into causes may include a fasting blood glucose to diagnose diabetes, thyroid function tests to diagnose hypothyroidism, and an ANA as an initial screen for scleroderma. ⊙

Discharge Planning:

Close follow-up with a primary care physician or diabetologist is essential for patients with frequent exacerbations of gastroparesis.

Patients with diabetes should review "sick day" instructions for diet and insulin management with a pharmacist or diabetes nurse prior to discharge.

Special Considerations:

Gastric pacemakers and pyloric injections of botulinum toxin are experimental therapies reserved for patients who do not respond to usual care.

In severe refractory cases, jejunal feeding through an endoscopic or surgically placed feeding tube may be considered. ⊙

References

American Gastroenterological Association technical review on the diagnosis and treatment of gastroparesis. *Gastroenterology* 127:1592–1622, 2004.

Maganti K, Onyemere K, Jones MP, et al: Oral erythromycin symptomatic relief of gastroparesis: A systematic review. *Am J Gastroenterol* 98:259–263, 2003.

4

Delirium

Delirium is defined as an acute alteration in consciousness with an inability to maintain attention, altered cognition, or perceptual disturbance. Patients may appear either sedated or hyperactive, and family members often notice delirium long before a physician would.

Delirium is a common presenting symptom of many underlying illnesses, particularly in the elderly.

The initial evaluation of a delirious patient focuses on finding the precipitating cause. Common precipitating causes include:

- Infection, especially pneumonia or urinary tract infection (UTI)
- Drugs, either prescribed or illicit
- Alcohol or benzodiazepine withdrawal
- Volume depletion and electrolyte abnormalities
- Thyroid disease
- Hypoxia
- Cardiac disease, including heart failure and ischemia

These orders are for a patient admitted with delirium attributed to a probable UTI.

Admit to: Medical Floor; Room Near the Nurses' Station Please

Most patients can be admitted to a medical floor, although some patients with delirium have an underlying cause requiring ICU care, such as sepsis or myocardial ischemia.

A Recommendation based on consistent and good quality patient-oriented evidence. **B** Recommendation based on inconsistent or limited quality patient-oriented evidence. **C** Recommendation based on usual practice, consensus, opinion, disease-oriented evidence, or case series for studies of diagnosis, treatment, and prevention of screening.

Some hospitals have a geriatric or delirium unit for patients admitted with or at high risk for confusion. These units have been effective in studies of multifactorial interventions to prevent or shorten the course of delirium. Many of the recommendations in this order set represent elements of published delirium interventions, although they appear to be more effective in prevention than in treatment of delirium. **Ⓐ**

A room near the nurses' station or in a high-traffic area allows multiple staff members to "keep an eye on" the patient.

D iagnosis: Delirium

C ondition: Guarded

Patients with delirium have a high 1-month mortality (14%), at least in part due to the severity of underlying illness. Patients with delirium also have longer hospital stays and prolonged (and sometimes incomplete) functional recovery compared with patients with similar underlying illness without delirium.

V ital Signs:

Routine. Check orthostatic vital signs on admit

The vital signs may provide clues to the cause of delirium: orthostasis suggests volume depletion, fever and tachycardia suggest infection, and low oxygen saturation suggests a pulmonary or cardiac cause.

A llergies: NKDA

A ctivity: Up to Chair for Meals. Ambulate with Assistance Each Shift. Fall Precautions

Patients with delirium are often impulsive and inattentive, placing them at high risk for falls. It is tempting to place them at bedrest to avoid injury, but normal activity should be maintained as long as it can be done fairly safely. **C**

N ursing:

Please ensure patient has hearing aids and glasses on during the day and has a clock or calendar in the room. Reorient patient frequently

Please assist patient to the bathroom q 2 hours while awake

Sensory deprivation appears to contribute to the development of delirium in the elderly. Patients should have (and be wearing) glasses or hearing aids when awake. The absence of clocks and calendars has also been associated with the development of delirium in already hospitalized patients. Single-intervention studies of any of these recommendations have not been done, but multicomponent interventions have been shown to decrease the incidence of delirium and the duration of delirium if it occurs. **A**

Foley catheters, IV lines, and other hospital paraphernalia should be avoided if possible because they decrease mobility and may worsen delirium.

Timed toileting can help avoid both incontinence and skin breakdown. **C**

Physical restraints should be avoided unless absolutely necessary to provide medical care or maintain patient safety. Applying restraints can turn confused but calm elderly patients into agitated and even more delirious patients. Family members or friends should be enlisted to stay in the patient's room to provide a familiar face and reorientation and to encourage the patient to stay in bed and leave IVs and so forth in place. **C**

D iet: General, Assist with Meal Set-Up

If the patient is not fully alert, his or her ability to swallow should be carefully assessed prior to allowing the patient to eat.

IV Fluids: None If Oral Intake Adequate. Heplock IV and Wrap with Protective Gauze

Volume depletion does appear to be the precipitating cause of some cases of delirium, and volume-depleted patients should of course receive IV fluid. However, if the patient is able to eat and drink, maintenance fluid should not be prescribed. Tubes and lines seem to increase agitation in delirious patients, and the struggle between nurse and patient to maintain an IV can escalate to physical restraints. If an IV is necessary, wrapping the IV site in Kerlix gauze or a special arm splint can help keep it in, particularly if it is heplocked. **C**

M edications:

Haloperidol 0.5–1 mg PO q 4 hours prn severe agitation
Trazodone 50 mg PO qhs
No **benzodiazepines or anticholinergic medications**
Amoxicillin-clavulanate 875 mg PO q 12 hours
Docusate 100 mg PO qd
Milk of magnesia 30 mL PO q 12 prn constipation
Heparin 5000 units SQ q 12 hours

Haloperidol is the most widely recommended drug for managing acute delirium, although there are limited data available from controlled trials. Prn doses should be reserved for significant agitation and disruptive behavior, not just confusion.

Trazodone at bedtime is less likely to have side effects than other drugs commonly prescribed for sleep. **C**

Many clinicians (and several small, uncontrolled trials) have found a low dose of quetiapine (e.g., 12.5 mg) to be effective in delirium, although there is much less experience with this drug than with Haldol. The sedating effect of quetiapine given at bedtime can help reset the deranged sleep/wake cycle of a delirious patient. **B**

Medications cause or contribute to an estimated one-third of cases of delirium, so the patient's medication list should be reviewed and any nonessential medications stopped, at least temporarily. The list of medications reported to cause delirium is long. Common culprits include benzodiazepines, opiates, corticosteroids, Parkinson's medications, anticholinergic drugs, digoxin, and quinolone antibiotics. **B**

Quinolones should be avoided in the elderly if other appropriate antibiotics are available, especially in patients who are already delirious. **C**

Benzodiazepines should not be used to manage delirium *unless* it is due to alcohol or sedative withdrawal. Then benzodiazepines are the agents of choice—*see* Alcohol Withdrawal, pp 220–225. **B**

Constipation could contribute to delirium and should be aggressively treated. **C**

If patients are not mobile, remember deep venous thrombosis (DVT) prophylaxis.

Labs and Diagnostic Studies:

Admit: Complete blood count (CBC), Chem 7, liver function tests, creatine kinase, myocardial bound (CK-MB), troponin, thyroid-stimulating hormone (TSH), digoxin level, urinalysis (UA), culture, chest x-ray (CXR), ECG

The admission labs are focused on establishing the cause of delirium. Elderly patients with UTIs or pneumonia may not have typical symptoms or signs, so a UA, culture, and CXR should be done in all. If suspicion for an infectious cause is high, blood cultures should be done as well.

Thyroid function tests and medication levels should be ordered in appropriate patients.

An ECG should be done to assess for cardiac ischemia. If the QT interval is prolonged, be very cautious in prescribing haloperidol because it may cause arrhythmia in this setting. **B**

D ischarge Planning:

The length of hospitalization depends on the underlying cause of delirium. Usually, it is not shorter than 3–4 days.

Social work, physical therapy, and occupational therapy should be consulted early in the stay for assistance with discharge planning. Patients may require a higher level of care than previously, at least temporarily.

A physician or pharmacist should carefully review the medication list, eliminating any that are unnecessary and ensuring the patient understands how the medications should be taken. A Medi-set and a large-type, accurate medication list at discharge may help.

If a patient admitted with delirium improves enough to be discharged home, consider a home safety evaluation.

S pecial Considerations:

Prevention of delirium is probably more effective than treatment. Intervention strategies should ideally target all elderly patients at high risk, including patients with preexisting dementia, those undergoing surgery, and those with long medication lists admitted with acute medical problems.

References

Al-Samarrai S, Dunn J, Newmark T, Gupta S: Quetiapine for treatment resistant delirium. *Psychosomatics* 44:350–351, 2003.

Milisen K, Lemiengre J, Braes T, Foreman MD: Multicomponent intervention strategies to manage delirium in hospitalized older people: Systematic review. *J Adv Nursing* 52:79–90, 2005.

Naughton B, Saltzman S, Ramadan F, et al: A multifactorial intervention to reduce prevalence of delirium and length of hospital stay. *JAGS* 53:18–23, 2005.

Practice Guideline for the Treatment of Patients with Delirium: The American Psychiatric Society. *Am J Psychiatry* 156S: 1–20, 1999.

Falls

Falls are a major problem in the elderly, annually affecting 35% of the older-than-65-years population and resulting in significant morbidity. Even elderly patients with a fall and a minor injury may be admitted with inadequate pain control, inadequate social support, or recurrent falls and concern for immediate home safety.

Falls in the elderly are often multifactorial. Common contributing factors include:

- Poor vision
- Poor footwear
- Poor strength or balance
- Polypharmacy
- Acute medical illness
- Orthostatic hypotension

These orders are for an 82-year-old man with hypertension and diabetes who fell to the ground in his home and was brought in by family for evaluation.

A dmit to: Floor, Room Near the Nurses' Station

D iagnosis: Falls

C ondition: Stable

V ital Signs:

Routine; check orthostatic vital signs on admission
   Orthostatic hypotension is a common contributing factor to falls in the elderly. It may be due to diabetic or other autonomic neuropathy or to medications. Orthostatics should be checked in all elderly patients presenting after a fall and considered positive if there is a > 20–30 mmHg drop in systolic blood pressure with standing.

A llergies: Routine

A ctivity: Ambulate with Assistance and Fall Precautions 3 × Daily

Although patients who have had a fall are at risk for another, prolonged bedrest will only worsen deconditioning and increase the risk of falls. Patients should be evaluated by a physical therapist and ambulate at least 2–3 times daily, with assistance and assistive devices as recommended by physical therapy (PT).

N ursing:

Fall precautions. Remind patient to sit at the edge of the bed for 3–5 minutes prior to standing
Assist to the toilet q 3 hours during the day
   Urinary urgency and a rush to the bathroom can contribute to falls. Timed toileting, whether in the hospital or at home, may be helpful.
   Especially for patients with orthostatic hypotension, sitting at the edge of the bed prior to standing can reduce the frequency of falls.

D iet: General

IV Fluids: None

No IV fluids are necessary if the patient is able to take oral fluids.

M edications:

Acetaminophen 650 mg PO q 6 hours, prn pain
Stop **the following outpatient meds: hydrochlorothiazide (HCTZ), amitriptyline, temazepam**
Vitamin D 800 IU PO qd
Calcium carbonate 1 g PO bid

Polypharmacy is a contributing factor to many falls: a medication list of more than four medications increases risk substantially in community-living elderly patients. As part of a multifactorial intervention, including exercise, home environment modification, and education, review, and alteration of medication lists reduced the risks for falls. **Ⓐ**

Specific medications to stop if possible:

- Psychotropic medications, including benzodiazepines, antipsychotics, sleeping aids, and antidepressants, especially tricyclics
- Diuretics, which can cause mild volume depletion and contribute to postural hypotension, as well as necessitate overly quick trips to the bathroom
- For patients with postural hypotension: antihypertensives, especially those that act predominantly as vasodilators (Mild supine hypertension may be better in the long run than recurrent falls resulting in injury. However, careful monitoring for severe supine hypertension should be continued and antihypertensives restarted if clearly necessary.)

Vitamin D supplementation can reduce the risk of both falls and fractures and should be prescribed for patients at risk.

Calcium supplementation should also be recommended because it is inexpensive and easy, although its benefit is not as clear.

Patients with documented osteoporosis and those with fractures associated with minimal trauma should also be treated with a bisphosphonate (after healing of any fracture). **Ⓐ**

L abs and Diagnostic Studies:

Admit: CBC, Chem 7, UA

Admit labs help screen for acute medical illness. Additional lab studies may be suggested by history and exam.

Plain films of any injured body part should also be done. If there is evidence of head trauma or the patient reports head injury, a CT scan of the head should be performed to rule out intracranial hemorrhage. **Ⓑ**

D ischarge Planning:

Social work should be consulted to assess the home situation and help the patient and family to choose the discharge destination—home versus a higher level of care.

Most patients who have suffered a fall without major injury can be discharged in 1–2 days, provided they are safe to return home. A PT and occupational therapy (OT) evaluation and appropriate assistive devices may prevent future falls. Outpatient PT for a strength and balance program can reduce the risk of falls. **Ⓑ**

A home safety evaluation reduces the risk of recurrent fall by about one-third. **Ⓐ**

A physician or pharmacist should review medications and eliminate inappropriate or unnecessary ones and provide an accurate list of discharge medications. **Ⓑ**

Hip protector pads reduce the risk of hip fracture in patients with falls and should be recommended at discharge for frail patients at persistent high risk of falls. **Ⓐ**

References

Kannus P, Sievanen H, Salvanen M, et al: Prevention of falls and consequent injuries in elderly people. *Lancet* 366:1885–1893, 2005.

Lin JT, Lane JM: Falls in the elderly population. *Phys Med Rehabil Med Clin North Am* 16:109–128, 2005.

Hip Fracture

Internists are involved in the care of almost every hip fracture patient, either as the attending physician of record or as a consultant. Although many patients with hip fracture are admitted to orthopedic surgeons, hip fractures are a disease of elderly patients, often with multiple comorbidities. The role of the internist is to advise the surgeon on timing of surgery and to prevent and manage complications. The internist should also investigate the mechanism of the fall and recommend further diagnostic or therapeutic intervention if indicated (*see* Falls, pp 122–126).

Admit to: Medical or Orthopedics Floor

Patients with hip fracture can be admitted to the floor unless concomitant disease, such as myocardial infarction (MI) or heart failure, requires admission to the ICU.

Diagnosis: Hip Fracture

C ondition: Guarded

Mortality of the initial hospitalization for hip fracture is 4%, but hip fracture has an even worse long-term prognosis from complications of the fracture or comorbid disease. One-year mortality after hip fracture is 25%. Only 60% of patients ambulatory before the fracture regain their prefracture walking ability at 6 months.

V ital Signs:

Every 4 hours

Tachycardia may be due to pain or to blood loss, especially when accompanied by hypotension.

Subtrochanteric hip fractures may be associated with substantial bleeding into the thigh muscles. Intertrochanteric and femoral neck fractures bleed much less because they are contained by the hip capsule.

A llergies: NKDA

A ctivity: Bedrest

Patients should be at bedrest until after the fracture is repaired. Then PT should be consulted for twice-daily sessions. The precautions in moving the operated hip will depend on the procedure done. ⊙

N ursing:

Place Foley catheter, monitor input and output (I/O), place oxygen at 2 L per nasal cannula if O$_2$ saturation < 92%, place sequential compression devices on both legs
Provide frequent reorientation, turn lights out, and limit interruptions at night. Call for any change in orientation

A Foley catheter is typically placed for skin care because the patient will be unable to get up or use a bedpan for several days.

Delirium is a major complication of hip fractures, usually beginning after but sometimes starting before surgery. Some nursing interventions may decrease the frequency or duration of delirium, including frequent reorientation, provision of clocks or calendars, and minimization of interruptions at night.

Bedside nurses may also pick up on delirium sooner than physicians, who see the patient for a much shorter time per day. If the nurse notes a change in mental status, take it seriously!

Diet: NPO for Operating Room (OR) in AM

The patient can eat if surgery will be delayed.

IV Fluids: D5 $\frac{1}{2}$ Normal Saline at 100 mL/h

Gentle hydration should be given when the patient is NPO because volume depletion may precipitate delirium. IV should be heplocked when taking PO well postoperatively.

Medications:

Warfarin 5 mg PO tonight
Acetaminophen 650 mg PO q 6 hours prn
Morphine 1–2 mg IV q 2 hours prn pain
Colace 250 mg PO qd
Senna 1 tablet PO bid
Calcium carbonate 2 tablets PO bid
Vitamin D 400 IU PO qd
Metoprolol 25 mg PO q 12 hours—hold for HR < 50 bpm,
   SBP < 100 mmHg
Cefazolin 1 g IV to accompany patient to the OR

Effective DVT prophylaxis is critical to the management of hip fracture. Enoxaparin, fondaparinux, or warfarin begun on the night before or night of surgery and continued postoperatively are all effective. Enoxaparin, however, should not be given within the 24 hours prior to an epidural catheter placement or with an epidural in place because of the risk of epidural hematoma. As many surgeons and anesthesiologists prefer to do hip fracture repair with epidural anesthesia, enoxaparin should not be given within 24 hours of the planned OR time. Fondiparinux is more expensive than the other two options. Ⓐ

Although many clinicians fear precipitating delirium with narcotics for hip fracture, uncontrolled pain can also lead to delirium. If a patient needs narcotics, use them. Especially after the fracture is fixed, many patients have surprisingly little pain and it is worth trying acetaminophen first. Ⓒ

A good bowel program is important as the patient will be receiving opiates and be at bedrest.

A hip fracture occurring with minor trauma, such as a fall, establishes the diagnosis of osteoporosis. The patient needs therapy to reduce the risk of future fractures. Ⓐ

Calcium and vitamin D may be started immediately, but bisphosphonates should not be given until after recovery because they may impair bone healing. Even if a patient was on estrogen or raloxifene for osteoporosis prior to admission, they should not be given because of the increased risk of DVT in a setting where the patient is already at high risk. Ⓑ

If the patient is felt to be at moderate or high risk of perioperative cardiac complications, it is appropriate to start a beta blocker and continue it through the perioperative period. If the patient is at low risk, a beta blocker may cause more complications than benefits and should be withheld. Ⓐ

Perioperative antibiotic prophylaxis should be administered within 60 minutes of incision time. Thus, they should not be started on the floor when the OR calls but go with the patient to preoperative holding. Ⓐ

Labs and Diagnostic Studies:

CBC with platelets, Chem 7, prothrombin time, partial thromboplastin time (PTT), ECG, type and cross for 2 units packed red blood cells (RBC), plain films of the left hip

Substantial blood loss may be seen with subtrochanteric fractures, less so with intertrochanteric or femoral neck fractures. Platelets and coagulation studies should be performed in preparation for surgery, in addition to a type and cross.

Plain films of the hip are very sensitive for hip fracture but rarely will not show an acute fracture. If clinical suspicion remains high, an MRI is a very sensitive test for fracture—if negative, fracture is ruled out.

ECG is performed as a preoperative baseline and to evaluate for any evidence of arrhythmia or cardiac disease that may have led to the fall.

Preoperative cardiac testing for ischemia is not indicated unless the patient has unstable angina or an acute MI. The outcome of hip fractures not treated surgically is poor, with persistent pain, inability to ambulate, and marked functional decline. Even patients with multiple medical problems are usually treated surgically. If clinical assessment indicates the patient is at moderate or high risk of perioperative cardiac complications, a beta blocker and close monitoring should be instituted. A noninvasive test for ischemia is likely to add little else to the management.

An echocardiogram should be performed if the history or physical exam suggests aortic stenosis, not because it would prevent surgery, but severe stenosis would alter anesthetic management.

Discharge Planning:

Social work consultation for skilled nursing facility (SNF) placement should be requested soon after admission because it is rare for a patient to be able to go home directly after hip fracture repair. ●

The patient should go to a SNF that is able to provide rehabilitation services, including daily PT and OT, to maximize the chance of regaining prior functional status and returning home. **C**

The patient should receive information about hip protectors, an inexpensive and not-too-bulky set of pads that can decrease the risk of hip fracture. **A**

The American College of Chest Physicians recommends DVT prophylaxis be continued for 28–35 days postoperatively because the risk of DVT and pulmonary embolism (PE) remains elevated long after hospital discharge. Warfarin is a less expensive option than enoxaparin, but a firm plan for international normalized ration (INR) monitoring should be in place before discharging a patient to a SNF on warfarin. If inadequate monitoring is available, enoxaparin may be a better, although more expensive, option. **B**

Although the patient will be discharged on calcium and vitamin D alone for osteoporosis, the primary care physician should institute bisphosphonate therapy after recovery. **C**

Special Considerations:

Surgical repair of hip fractures should be performed within the first 24–48 hours after fracture unless an medical problem requires stabilization. Observational studies show an increase in complications and mortality when surgery is performed later, although some delays may be due to sicker patients. **B**

References

Bitsch M, Foss N, Kristensen B, Kehlet H: Pathogenesis and management strategies for postoperative delirium after hip fracture. *Acta Orthop Scand* 75(4):378–389, 2004.

Kessel B: Hip fracture prevention in postmenopausal women. *Obstet Gynecol Surv* 59(6):446–455, 2004.

Morris AH, Zuckerman AD: Improving the continuum of care for patients with hip fracture. *J Bone Joint Surg* 84:670–674, 2002.

Morrison RS, Chassin MR, Siu AL: The medical consultant's role in caring for patients with hip fracture. *Ann Intern Med* 128:1010–1020, 1998.

Cancer, Admit for Chemotherapy

Patients admitted for chemotherapy have diverse needs depending on the type of primary tumor, extent of disease, and overall health status. Many chemotherapy regimens can be given in outpatient infusion centers, but high-dose regimens are still typically administered in the hospital because they are more complex and more likely to cause complications.

Complications of outpatient chemotherapy, such as mucositis, anemia, and thrombocytopenia, may also lead to admission.

In most hospitals, oncologists are responsible for writing orders for chemotherapy. Orders for supportive care are reviewed here.

Admit to: Floor, Private Room

Most patients will be admitted to the oncology ward, and neutropenic patients should have a private room to reduce the risk of infection.

Diagnosis: Cancer, Admit for Chemotherapy

Condition: Stable

Patients admitted for chemotherapy are generally stable at the time of admission but are at risk for severe complications over the course of their stay.

A Recommendation based on consistent and good quality patient-oriented evidence. **B** Recommendation based on inconsistent or limited quality patient-oriented evidence. **C** Recommendation based on usual practice, consensus, opinion, disease-oriented evidence, or case series for studies of diagnosis, treatment, and prevention of screening.

V ital Signs:
Routine

A llergies: Routine

A ctivity: Encourage Activity with Assistance, Fall Precautions

Patients with chemotherapy-induced thrombocytopenia are at risk for intracranial hemorrhage and other severe injuries with falls. ☉

N ursing:
Guaiac stools, neurologic checks q 4 hours. No IM injections if platelets < 50,000/mm^3. Call for any temperature > 37.9°C
Oral care q shift

Nursing orders should include monitoring for complications of chemotherapy. Severe thrombocytopenia may cause spontaneous bleeding in the central nervous system (CNS), gastrointestinal (GI) tract, or elsewhere.

Fever should be addressed immediately in neutropenic patients. Management of neutropenic fever is reviewed in Febrile Neutropenia, pp 137–142. ☉

D iet: No Unpeeled Fresh Fruits or Fresh Vegetables

Patients with chemotherapy-induced neutropenia are at risk for infection with environmental fungi. Fruits and vegetables should be either peeled or cooked to reduce that risk. ☉

IV Fluids: None If Adequate Oral Intake

Prehydration with IV fluid is a common component of chemotherapy, and appropriate IV fluids are typically ordered by the oncologist. Aggressive hydration is prescribed for patients at risk of tumor lysis syndrome.

Nausea and vomiting is increasingly uncommon with modern antiemetic regimens. However, if nausea and vomiting occurs and persists, maintenance IV fluids should be prescribed.

Total parenteral nutrition (TPN) may be necessary if the patient develops severe mucositis with inability to eat or cancer cachexia.

Medications:

Filgrastim (granulocyte colony stimulating factor [G-CSF])
   300 μg SQ qd (increase dose to 480 μg for patients > 70 kg)
Prophylactic antiemetics

- Ondansetron (Zofran) 16 mg PO prechemotherapy
- Dexamethasone 12 mg IV pretherapy, 8 mg PO qd days 2–4

Prn antiemetics

- Prochlorperazine (Compazine) 10 mg IV/PO q 6 hours prn nausea
- Metoclopramide (Reglan) 10 mg IV/PO q 6 hours prn nausea
- Dronabinol (THC or Marinol) 2.5–10 mg PO q 6 hours prn
- Lorazepam (Ativan): 0.5–2 mg IV/PO q 6 hours prn nausea

Magic Mouthwash (viscous lidocaine + Benadryl + Maalox)
   15 mL swish and spit q 2 hours prn mouth pain
Cetacaine spray prn mouth pain
Baclofen 5–10 mg PO of 8 hours prn hiccups
Docusate 250 mg PO bid and/or senna 2 tablets PO qhs
Bisacodyl 5–10 mg PO qd prn constipation

Colony-stimulating factors, such as G-CSF, should not be given routinely but should be reserved for patients with a prior episode of febrile neutropenia or a > 40% risk of febrile neutropenia. Patients older than age 70 years receiving moderately bone marrow–suppressive chemotherapy regimens and all adult patients receiving highly marrow-suppressive regimens should be treated beginning 24 hours after first chemotherapy dose and continuing until neutrophil count is > 1500/mm^3 on two consecutive days, for a maximum of 14 days. **Ⓐ**

The antiemetic regimen is dictated by the chemotherapy regimen. Some, such as cisplatin-based regimens, cause vomiting in most patients and require aggressive prophylaxis with a 5HT 3 receptor antagonist, such as ondansetron *plus* dexamethasone. Less emetogenic regimens require prophylaxis with less expensive medications, such as dexamethasone or prochlorperazine, whereas the lowest-risk patients need only *prn* antiemetics. For current clinical practice guidelines, *see* References, p 137.

Mucositis can be a major complication of chemotherapy, causing severe pain and poor nutrition. Treatment is primarily symptomatic. A mixture of viscous lidocaine and Maalox, Cetacaine spray (a topical anesthetic), or sucralfate slurry may be used. **Ⓒ**

The majority of hospitalized cancer patients develop constipation related to narcotics, dehydration, inactivity, or other factors. All cancer patients should receive prophylactic therapy against constipation. Suppositories and enemas should not be used to treat constipation in neutropenic patients due to the risk of perirectal abscess. **Ⓒ**

Ⓛ abs and Diagnostic Studies:

Complete blood count (CBC) with platelets, Chem 7 daily

Daily labs are performed to monitor for bone marrow suppression and electrolyte abnormalities.

Patients with cancers with high cell turnover (e.g., some leukemias and lymphomas, and bulky tumors) are also at risk for tumor lysis syndrome with the initiation of chemotherapy and require more frequent lab monitoring. Cells die and lyse rapidly, releasing large amounts of potassium, phosphate, and uric acid, leading to arrhythmias, severe hypocalcemia, and renal failure. These patients need to have a Chem 7, calcium, phosphate, and uric acid level checked every 6 hours with initial therapy. ❽

Discharge Planning:

Patients should be ambulating, able to keep up with nutritional support, and afebrile before release.

Special Considerations:

Because of the high risk of complications with chemotherapeutic agents, oncologists are usually responsible for writing chemotherapy orders.

References

Practice Guidelines in Oncology: Antiemesis: www.nccn.org/professionals/physician_gls/PDF/antiemesis.pdf; accessed 8/21/05.

Practice Guidelines in Oncology: Myeloid growth factors: www.nccn.org/professionals/physician_gls/PDF/myeloid_growth.pdf; accessed 8/21/05.

Febrile Neutropenia

Neutropenic fever is defined as a single temperature $\geq 38.3°C$, or a temperature $\geq 38°C$ for 1 hour, with a neutrophil count of $< 500/mm^3$. Most patients with neutropenic fever should be admitted to the hospital for close observation and treatment because they are at high risk for occult bacterial infections and mortality. Very carefully selected low-risk patients at experienced centers may be treated as outpatients, provided they have 24-hour access to medical care. *See* References, p 142 for IDSA clinical practice guidelines with further information on selecting low-risk patients for outpatient therapy. **Ⓐ**

Unusual sites of infection should be considered in neutropenic patients. Vascular access device infections, perirectal abscesses, sinusitis, typhlitis (inflammation of the cecum, typically presenting with abdominal pain), and oral infections should not be overlooked. **Ⓒ**

Ⓐdmit to: Floor—Single Room

Neutropenic patients should have a single room to reduce exposure to infection.

Patients with neutropenic fever may prevent with severe sepsis, in which case ICU admission is indicated.

Ⓓiagnosis: Febrile Neutropenia

Ⓒondition: Serious

Historically, neutropenic patients with fever had up to 70% mortality, most due to infection. Now, with close observation and early initiation of broad-spectrum antibiotics, survival is > 90%.

Ⓥital Signs:

Routine. Check temperature q 4 hours

Ⓐllergies: NKDA

Activity: Encourage Activity with Assistance. Fall Precautions

Patients with chemotherapy-induced thrombocytopenia are at risk for intracranial hemorrhage and other severe injuries with falls. ◉

Nursing:

Guaiac stools, neurologic checks q 4 hours. No IM injections if platelets < 50,000/mm^3. Call for any temperature > 37.9°C
Oral care q shift

Nursing orders should include monitoring for other complications of chemotherapy. Severe thrombocytopenia may cause spontaneous bleeding in the CNS, GI tract, or elsewhere.

Diet: No Unpeeled Fresh Fruits or Fresh Vegetables

Patients with chemotherapy-induced neutropenia are at risk for infection with environmental fungi. Fruits and vegetables should be either peeled or cooked to reduce that risk. ◉

IV Fluids: None If Adequate Oral Intake

Patients with persistent high fever may require IV fluids because of insensible fluid losses, often coupled with poor PO intake. ◉

Medications:

Imipenem 500 mg IV q 6 hours

Initial empiric antibiotics should broadly cover Gram-positive and Gram-negative pathogens (including *Pseudomonas*) and should also include appropriate coverage for suspected sites of infection (e.g., catheter exit site infection).

In the absence of localizing signs and symptoms, any of the following antibiotic regimens may be used: ❶

- Ceftazidime 2 g IV q 8 hours
- Imipenem 500 mg IV q 6 hours
- Meropenem
- Cefepime 2 g IV q 8 hours
- Aminoglycoside plus antipseudomonal penicillin or cephalosporin *or* a carbapenem

Subsequent antibiotic therapy is guided by culture results, localization of infection, duration of fever, and duration of neutropenia. *See* References, p 142 for the clinical practice guidelines with further information.

Vancomycin should be added to the initial empiric antibiotic regimen for patients with: ❸

- Hypotension or cardiovascular compromise
- Clinically suspected intravascular catheter infection
- Mucositis
- Known colonization or prior infection with methicillin-resistant *Staphylococcus aureus*
- Can be considered for patients who were on prophylactic quinolone prior to the development of fever

Myeloid growth factors (i.e., G-CSF) have not been shown to improve outcomes in patients with neutropenic fever but are generally recommended for high-risk patients to shorten the duration of neutropenia: patients with invasive fungal infection, pneumonia, and progressive infection despite antibiotics. ❸

L abs and Diagnostic Studies:

Admit: CBC with differential, Chem 7, liver function tests, blood cultures × 2, urinalysis (UA) and culture, chest x-ray (CXR) posteroanterior (PA) and lateral

Daily: CBC with differential, Chem 7. Repeat blood cultures q 24 hours if febrile

Daily labs are performed to monitor the degree of bone marrow suppression and electrolyte imbalance. ●

Liver function tests and UA should be performed at admission to assess the site of infection. ●

CXR should be performed if the patient has any respiratory symptom or sign or if outpatient therapy is being considered. ●

Two blood cultures should be performed, at least one of which should come from the indwelling line, if present. To maximize yield, 20–40 mL of blood should be used for each culture. ⓑ

Other studies should be guided by clinical presentation, results of initial laboratories, and response to initial therapy.

D ischarge Planning:

The duration of hospitalization will depend on the cause of fever, the severity of illness, and the anticipated time to recovery of neutrophil counts. Some low-risk patients may be discharged on oral antibiotics after a brief initial period of hospitalization, with careful outpatient follow-up. Patients with documented infection and those with longer anticipated periods of neutropenia will usually be hospitalized until counts recover and fever has resolved.

S pecial Considerations:

Neutropenic patients may have a blunted inflammatory response to infection and are thus treated with antibiotics even when no documented source of fever is found. A patient with pneumonia may have no change on CXR. A patient with cellulitis may have only very subtle skin findings. Clinical disease may initially appear to worsen as counts recover, as the local inflammatory response improves.

References

IDSA 2002 guidelines for the use of antimicrobial agents in neutropenic patients with cancer. *Clin Infect Dis* 34:730–751, 2002.

Practice Guidelines in Oncology: Fever and neutropenia: www.nccn.org/professionals/physician_gls/PDF/fever.pdf; accessed 8/21/05.

Bacterial Endocarditis

The diagnosis of endocarditis may not be obvious on admission. It may take several days for a pathogen to be isolated. However, endocarditis should be considered in patients with fever and a heart murmur, especially if embolic phenomena or a history of IV drug use is present.

Patients with a prosthetic valve and fever should be strongly suspected of having endocarditis until an alternate source of fever is clearly diagnosed.

A dmit to: Telemetry

Telemetry allows for monitoring of conduction disturbances and arrhythmias that could signal the presence of myocardial abscess or worsening heart failure.

Patients with hemodynamic instability require ICU care.

D iagnosis: Bacterial Endocarditis

C ondition: Serious

V ital Signs:

Temperature, BP, pulse, RR, and oxygen saturation q 4 hours until afebrile for 24 hours, then per routine

Pay careful attention to hypotension because it may be a sign of worsening valvular insufficiency or cardiac failure.

A Recommendation based on consistent and good quality patient-oriented evidence. **B** Recommendation based on inconsistent or limited quality patient-oriented evidence. **C** Recommendation based on usual practice, consensus, opinion, disease-oriented evidence, or case series for studies of diagnosis, treatment, and prevention of screening.

A llergies: Cephalosporins Cause Rash

A ctivity: As Tolerated

The degree of hemodynamic compromise will dictate the appropriate level of activity. ⊙

N ursing:

Daily weights
Strict input and output (I/O)

D iet: Regular

If heart failure is present, prescribe a low-sodium diet. ⊙

If hemodynamic compromise is present and urgent surgery may be needed, make the patient NPO except medications.

IV Fluids: As Needed

M edications:

Vancomycin 1 g IV q 12 hours
Gentamicin 1 mg/kg IV q 8 hours
Tylenol 325–650 mg PO q 4–6 hours as needed for fever; not to exceed 4 g in 24 hours (or 2 g in 24 hours if end-stage liver disease)

The choice of antibiotic depends on the suspected organism. The most common pathogens are *Staphylococci*, *Streptococci*, and *Enterococcus*. Empiric antibiotic coverage with vancomycin and gentamicin should be replaced with tailored antibiotic therapy once culture results are available. ⊙

If infection with methicillin-resistant *Staphylococcus aureus* is *not* a concern, then nafcillin (a bacteriocidal agent) 2 g IV q 4 hours should be substituted in the empiric regimen for vancomycin (a bacteriostatic agent). ⊙

In patients with prosthetic valves, rifampin 600 mg PO qd should be added empirically. ⊙

Consider consultation from an infectious disease specialist when selecting an antimicrobial regimen and duration of treatment. ⊙

L abs and Diagnostic Studies:

Admission: Blood cultures × 3 (from different sites); complete blood count (CBC) with differential; Chem 7; liver function tests (LFTs); urinalysis (UA); posteroanterior (PA) and lateral chest x-ray (CXR); ECG; echocardiogram

Daily: CBC until white blood count (WBC) normalized; Chem 7 while on antibiotics that can affect renal function

Blood cultures are key to diagnosis and should be obtained before antibiotics are given whenever possible. If blood cultures are positive, a follow-up culture should be done daily until the bacteremia clears. ⊙

If HACEK or other fastidious organisms are suspected, ask the microbiology lab to hold the blood cultures for 21 days. If cultures fail to reveal a pathogen and endocarditis is still suspected, consider sending serology for organisms such as *Brucella, Bartonella,* and *Coxiella burnetii.*

LFTs may show evidence of transaminitis in the setting of embolic phenomena to the liver. Hematuria on UA may indicate glomerulonephritis. CXR may show evidence of emboli in the setting of right-sided endocarditis or volume overload in the setting of left ventricular failure from mitral or aortic valve disease.

The ECG should be examined for evidence of conduction delay. The presence of atrioventricular (AV) nodal or bundle branch block suggests the possibility of myocardial abscess that may require urgent surgical intervention. The ECG should be followed daily at first to assess for new conduction abnormalities. ⊙

Echocardiography is usually needed for diagnosis and to assess the degree of valvular disease and ventricular function. Transesophageal echocardiogram (which is more sensitive for vegetations, abscesses, and perivalvular leaks) should be obtained in patients with suspected perivalvular abscess, in patients with prosthetic valves, and in patients with suboptimal echocardiographic windows. **Ⓐ**

In other patients, transthoracic echocardiography is a reasonable first test. If a transthoracic echocardiogram is negative and the clinical suspicion for endocarditis remains moderate to high, a transesophageal echocardiogram should be obtained. **Ⓐ**

The lab and other tests described previously, plus a careful history and exam, will provide the information needed in most cases to determine whether a patient meets diagnostic criteria (i.e., Duke's criteria) for the diagnosis of infective endocarditis (Table 1).

Discharge Planning:

Plan early for the possibility of prolonged IV antibiotics (4–6 weeks) if endocarditis is confirmed. Options may include home IV infusion, outpatient IV antibiotics at an infusion center, or nursing home placement.

Special Considerations:

Cardiac surgery consultation should be obtained early in any patient with evidence of heart failure, myocardial abscess, systemic emboli with residual large valvular vegetation, inability to clear blood cultures with antibiotics alone, or infection with fungi or untreatable pathogens. **Ⓑ**

Infectious disease and cardiology consultants should be considered for assistance with initial management, including choice of antibiotics and management of any cardiac complications.

Table 1 Modified Duke Criteria for Diagnosis of Infective Endocarditis*

Major Criteria

Typical microorganism (e.g., *Staphylococcus aureus*, streptococci) grown from 2 blood cultures

Any microorganism grown from persistently positive blood cultures

Positive serologic test or single positive blood culture for *Coxiella burnetii* (Q fever)

Echocardiogram showing oscillating intracardiac mass, abscess, or new dehiscence of prosthetic valve

Physical exam showing new valvular regurgitation (change in preexisting murmur not sufficient)

Minor Criteria

Predisposing heart condition or injection drug use

Fever >38.0°C

Vascular phenomena (e.g., major arterial emboli, septic pulmonary infarcts, mycotic aneurysm, intracranial hemorrhage, conjunctival hemorrhages, Janeway lesions [petechiae or splinter hemorrhages not sufficient])

Immunologic phenomena (e.g., glomerulonephritis, Osler nodes, Roth spots, positive rheumatoid factor)

Serologic evidence of infection or positive blood cultures not meeting a major criterion

Diagnosis

Definite endocarditis: either 2 major, 1 major plus 3 minor, or 5 minor criteria

Possible endocarditis: either 1 major plus 1 minor or 3 minor criteria

*Adapted from Li JS, Sexton DJ, et al. Proposed modifications to the Duke criteria for the diagnosis of infective endocarditis. *Clin Infect Dis* 30:633–8, 2000.

References

Baddour LM, Wilson WR, Bayer AS, et al: Infective endocarditis: Diagnosis, antimicrobial therapy, and management of complications: A statement for healthcare professionals from the Committee on Rheumatic Fever, Endocarditis, and Kawasaki Disease, Council on Cardiovascular Disease in the Young, and the Councils on Clinical Cardiology, Stroke, and Cardiovascular Surgery and Anesthesia, American Heart Association—executive summary: Endorsed by the Infectious Diseases Society of America. *Circulation* 111:3167–3184, 2005.

Gilbert D, Moellering RC, Eliopoulos GM, Sande M: *The Sanford Guide to Antimicrobial Therapy.* Hyde Park, VT, Antimicrobial Therapy, Inc., 2005.

Li JS, Sexton DJ, Mick N, et al: Proposed modifications to the Duke criteria for the diagnosis of infective endocarditis. *Clin Infect Dis* 30:633–638, 2000.

Moreillon P, Yok-Ai Q: Infective endocarditis. *Lancet* 363:139–149, 2004.

Mylonakis E, Calderwood SB: Infective endocarditis. *N Engl J Med* 345:1318–1330, 2001.

Cellulitis

Patients with cellulitis can often be managed as outpatients with oral antibiotics. Consider admission for:

- Signs of systemic toxicity or concern for rapidly progressing infection
- Patients unable to keep leg affected by cellulitis elevated
- Patients unable to tolerate oral antibiotics

In cellulitis with abscess, admit the patient who requires initial assistance with dressing changes following incision and drainage.

Necrotizing fasciitis is a much more severe and urgent soft tissue infection, and suspicion of this diagnosis requires admission and urgent surgical consultation for débridement.

These orders are for a 38-year-old woman with obesity and tinea pedis, presenting with fever, nausea, and cellulitis of the right leg with a small abscess that has been drained.

A dmit to: Floor

Most patients with cellulitis are clinically stable and can be admitted to the floor.

Rare patients with sepsis syndrome or suspected necrotizing fasciitis should be admitted to the ICU, with prompt surgical consultation.

D iagnosis: Cellulitis

C ondition: Stable

Most patients with cellulitis are stable. If hemodynamically unstable, consider an alternate, more aggressive process such as necrotizing fasciitis or unusual organisms such as *Clostridium* sp. or *Vibrio* sp.

V ital Signs:

Routine

A llergies: NKDA

A ctivity: Elevate Affected Area When in Bed

Elevation reduces swelling and may help cellulitis resolve more quickly.

N ursing:

Dress abscess wounds with twice-daily wet-to-dry dressings

Deep abscess cavities need to be packed to prevent the wound from closing before the infection is completely resolved. Patients should be taught to do dressing changes because dressings will continue after discharge.

Diet: Regular

IV Fluids: Heplock IV

Maintenance fluids should be given if the patient is unable to take oral fluids.

Medications:

Cefazolin 1.5 g IV q 8 hours
Ibuprofen 600 mg PO q 8 hours
Oxycodone 5–10 mg PO q 4 hours prn pain
Spectazole cream to both feet once daily

Because streptococci and staphylococci cause most cellulitis, first-generation cephalosporins are typically prescribed for patients at low risk for methicillin-resistant *S. aureus* (MSSA). When the patient is ready for discharge, cephalexin may be substituted for cefazolin. **Ⓐ**

Nafcillin and oxacillin are alternatives for MSSA.

For patients with penicillin allergy, clindamycin may be substituted. **Ⓑ**

Vancomycin 1 g IV q 12 hours, linezolid, or daptomycin should be prescribed for inpatients with prior methicillin-resistant *S. aureus* (MRSA) or those at high risk for MRSA. Populations at high risk for MRSA include IV drug users, jail inmates, residents of long-term care facilities, homosexual men, and health care contacts including recent surgery, dialysis, or other indwelling devices. **Ⓐ**

Trimethoprim-sulfamethoxazole DS 2 tablets PO bid or doxycycline can be prescribed for patients at high risk of MRSA at discharge, after clinical improvement with vancomycin. **Ⓑ**

Effective pain control often decreases extent of symptoms and hospital stay. In one small randomized study, nonsteroidal anti-inflammatory drugs (NSAIDs) also decreased time to clinical improvement. Schedule NSAIDs for pain control, except in patients with renal insufficiency or gastrointestinal (GI) intolerance. ❸

Consider narcotics if NSAIDs provide inadequate relief of pain. ❻

Tinea pedis is an important predisposing factor for cellulitis—breaks in the skin caused by the fungal infection allow bacterial pathogens to enter. Consider treatment with topical antifungal cream such as Spectazole or an oral antifungal. This is especially important in patients with diabetes, who are at risk for more severe complications, including amputation, with cellulitis.

Labs and Diagnostic Studies:

CBC, Chem 7, blood cultures × 2

The diagnosis of cellulitis should be based on suggestive history and exam findings. Elevated WBC provides support for diagnosis, but patients with cellulitis may have a normal WBC.

Blood cultures are positive in < 5% of patients with cellulitis. Draw cultures in patients with systemic toxicity, immunosuppression, therapeutic nonresponse, unusual exposures such as bites or water exposure, or recurrent infection. ❻

Imaging is not necessary in most patients with cellulitis but can be helpful in certain situations. Ultrasound can help localize occult abscesses and facilitate drainage. Plain films are useful if gas-producing organisms are suspected; for example, if on physical exam there is crepitus, bullae, blistering, or other unusual findings. ❸

If necrotizing fasciitis is suspected, obtain surgical consultation before imaging—immediate exploratory surgery is the standard of care. More extensive labs and immediate broad-spectrum antibiotics are also necessary.

Discharge Planning:

Erythema may worsen within the first 24–48 hours of treatment but should improve after that time. Patients may be discharged when taking oral medication and fever and erythema are reduced, or if the patient is reliable for an early follow-up appointment. Patients who have had one episode of cellulitis are at markedly increased risk of having another.

Discharge education should include measures to reduce the incidence of cellulitis, such as moisturization of the feet, treatment of tinea pedis, and treatment of edema, with leg elevation, compression hose, and if appropriate, diuretics.

Special Considerations:

Necrotizing fasciitis, a disease that may be mistaken for simple cellulitis, progresses rapidly and can be fatal—emergent surgical consultation is warranted. Clues to the diagnosis of necrotizing fasciitis are:

- Severe tenderness upon palpation of infected area
- Numbness of the area
- Rapid worsening of erythema and pain
- History of injection drug use (IDU)
- WBC > 20,000 cells/mm^3
- Low serum sodium

Orbital cellulitis is an ophthalmologic emergency. Carefully evaluate patients with facial cellulitis for involvement of the orbit. If extraocular movements are impaired, obtain an orbital CT scan and consult ophthalmology immediately.

If a patient with hand cellulitis has any loss of hand function, an orthopedic surgeon should be consulted immediately.

Cellulitis associated with human or animal bites has a different range of pathogens—if the patient requires admission, ampicillin-sulbactam would be an appropriate initial antibiotic choice.

References

Bisno AL, Stevens DL: Streptococcal infections of skin and soft tissues. *N Engl J Med* 334:240–245, 1996.

Dall L, Peterson S, Simmons T, Dall A: Rapid resolution of cellulitis in patients managed with combination antibiotic and antiinflammatory therapy. *Cutis* 75:177–180, 2005.

Stevens DL, Bisno AL, Chambers HF, et al: Practice guidelines for the management of skin and soft tissue infections. *Clin Infect Dis* 41:1373–1406, 2005.

Swartz MN: Cellulitis. *N Engl J Med* 350:904–912, 2004.

Fever in Injection Drug Use

Patients with a history of injection drug (IDU) use are frequently admitted with infectious complications. Because clinical and initial lab evaluation cannot reliably exclude endocarditis, and because follow-up may be unreliable, some hospitals admit all patients with a history of IDU and unexplained fever. **B**

Common infections in injection drug users include cellulitis, abscesses, and pneumonia. Less common conditions that should not be missed include necrotizing fasciitis, epidural abscess, septic arthritis, pyomyositis, tuberculosis (TB), hepatitis, and acute HIV.

These orders are for a 28-year-old woman with a history of IDU who presents with fever.

A dmit to: Floor

A new regurgitant murmur, embolic signs of endocarditis, and conduction abnormalities on ECG strongly suggest acute bacterial endocarditis. However, none of these findings is sensitive enough to *exclude* endocarditis if absent. If endocarditis is strongly suspected, the patient should be admitted to a telemetry floor for continuous monitoring.

D iagnosis: Fever in IDU

C ondition: Stable

If endocarditis is strongly suspected, condition may be "guarded."

V ital Signs:

Routine, with temperature q 4 hours

A llergies: NKDA

Activity: Ad lib in room. Patient should remain in isolation until MRSA is excluded

MRSA is increasing in prevalence, especially among IDU. Most hospitals restrict contact between patients with MRSA and other patients. Patients should wash hands and don a gown and gloves prior to leaving the room for necessary tests or procedures. ◐

N ursing:

Please review visitor policy and smoking policy with patient
Assess pain q 4 hours
Monitor for sedation, and call physician if this occurs

Patients with active IDU are often challenging for physicians and nursing staff. Clear, consistent, and nonjudgmental communication about the hospital's policy on visitors, smoking, and illicit substance use and careful attention to pain management may help to avoid conflict.

A formal behavioral contract outlining the goals of care, physician responsibility, and patient responsibilities, as well as consequences for nonadherence to rules, may be useful in some cases.

D iet: General

IV Fluids: None

Patients with persistent high fever may have large insensible fluid losses and require IV fluids, especially if they are unable to drink oral fluids. Other patients do not require IV fluid if able to take fluid PO.

M edications:

Methadone 30 mg PO q 12 hours—hold for sedation. May increase to 40 mg PO q 12 hours if patient reports inadequate control of withdrawal symptoms and has no evidence of sedation
Oxycodone 15–30 mg PO q 4 hours prn pain
Ibuprofen 600 mg PO tid
Nicotine patch 21 mg transdermal daily

Antibiotic selection should be guided by the likely site of infection and suspected organisms. If a patient with IDU and fever has no localizing signs or symptoms and is clinically stable, antibiotics may be withheld pending cultures. However, if endocarditis is suspected, empiric therapy should be initiated. *See* Bacterial Endocarditis, pp 143–148.

In many communities, the prevalence of MRSA is high enough in injection drug users that initial therapy for cellulitis targets MRSA. Those with less severe cellulitis may be treated with oral regimens for MRSA, including trimethoprim-sulfamethoxazole (TMP-SMX) and doxycycline. **B**

Management of withdrawal symptoms and pain are crucial to the care of patients with active opiate use. Methadone 30 mg every 12 hours is an appropriate starting dose for most patients, but the dose should be decreased for very thin patients or those with renal or hepatic insufficiency. The dose should be increased for inadequate control of withdrawal symptoms, as long as the patient is *not* sedated. **C**

Opiate-dependent patients exhibit tolerance to all narcotics and will need higher-than-average doses of narcotic analgesics to control pain. NSAIDs may be a useful adjunct in treating pain.

Nicotine dependence often accompanies IDU, and withdrawal can make hospitalization even more difficult for these patients. A nicotine patch can alleviate these symptoms.

Labs and Diagnostic Studies:

CBC, Chem 7, LFTs, blood cultures × 2, CXR. Hepatitis A and B serologies, HIV serology

At least two sets of blood cultures should be performed to exclude bacteremia and endocarditis. Ideally, three sets should be done, but limited IV access is frequently a problem in this patient population. In one series, one of the first two blood cultures was positive in 98% of bacteremic patients with a history of IDU. *However,* street antibiotic use is common in IDU, and patients with endocarditis may have negative cultures if they have recently taken oral antibiotics. In the absence of antibiotic use, two to three negative blood cultures argue strongly against a diagnosis of endocarditis. **B**

CXR should be performed unless there is an obvious source of fever, such as cellulitis, on exam. Pneumonia is a common cause of fever in this patient population, and the CXR may provide clues to underlying endocarditis, such as septic emboli or evidence of pulmonary edema. **C**

An echocardiogram should be performed if endocarditis is strongly suspected based on clinical findings *or* positive blood cultures. Patients with a history of IDU and another obvious source of fever do not require an echo to "rule out endocarditis." **ⓒ**

Because this patient population often has limited access to health care, hospitalization offers an opportunity to provide some primary care. If hepatitis A and B vaccines have not been given, check serologies and administer vaccine if negative. If the patient has not had recent HIV testing and consents to testing in the hospital, it should also be considered. **ⓒ**

Discharge Planning:

Social work should be consulted early in the hospitalization of all injection drug users. Information about methadone maintenance programs, Narcotics Anonymous, and community support services may help the patient to break the cycle of addiction, infection, and hospitalization. This patient population often has limited financial resources, so social work can help with arrangements for discharge medications and follow-up. Prior to discharge, the patient should also receive education about clean needles and needle exchange programs, which reduce the risk of bacterial and HIV infection. **ⓒ**

Reference

Gordon RJ, Lowy FD: Bacterial infections in drug users. *N Engl J Med* 353:1945–1954, 2005.

Meningitis

Patients with meningitis typically present with fever, headache, neck stiffness, or confusion. Meningitis may be caused by bacterial or viral (or, less commonly, fungal) pathogens, or by noninfectious causes such as drugs or collagen vascular disease.

In immunocompetent adults, the most common causative organisms are *Streptococcus pneumoniae, Neisseria meningitides, Listeria monocytogenes,* and *Haemophilus influenza.* Patients with recent neurosurgery or head trauma may have Gram-negative rod meningitis.

All patients with suspected bacterial meningitis should be admitted to the hospital for IV antibiotics and close observation. These orders are for a 62-year-old woman with suspected bacterial meningitis.

Admit to: ICU, Droplet Precautions

Most patients with meningitis are admitted to a medical or neurology ICU, with very close observation. Patients with a normal level of consciousness and vital signs may be admitted to the floor if very close monitoring and frequent neurologic checks are available. Patients with sepsis syndrome, seizures, or decreased level of consciousness must be admitted to the ICU.

Patients should be placed in droplet precautions until meningococcal meningitis is ruled out, to prevent nosocomial transmission of the disease.

Diagnosis: Meningitis

Condition: Guarded

Despite effective antibiotic therapy, the mortality rate for adults with bacterial meningitis remains high, up to 25%. Long-term complications are also common among survivors.

V ital Signs:

Every 4 hours, with neurologic checks q 2 hours × 24 hours
Neurologic status should be monitored carefully, and decreasing level of consciousness should prompt reevaluation and transfer to the ICU.

A llergies: NKDA

Activity: Bedrest for the first 24 hours, then mobilize as tolerated

N ursing:

Fall precautions. Call for temperature > 38.5°C, HR > 110 bpm, SBP < 100 mmHg, changing neurologic status
Increasing HR or falling BP should prompt immediate reevaluation for the development of sepsis syndrome.

D iet: NPO for Now. Please Assess Ability to Swallow Safely in AM

Patients who are fully alert can eat a general diet. Those with any change in level of consciousness should be NPO until the safety of swallowing is evaluated, to avoid aspiration.

IV Fluids: D5 ½ Normal Saline (NS) at 100 mL/h. Heplock if PO Intake Adequate

M edications:

Dexamethasone 0.15 mg/kg IV now, then q 6 hours. First dose must be given along with antibiotics
Ceftriaxone 2 g IV q 12 hours, first dose now
Vancomycin 1 g IV q 12 hours, first dose now
Ampicillin 2 g IV q 6 hours, first dose now
Dexamethasone decreases morbidity and mortality in adults with *S. pneumonia,* the leading cause of meningitis

in adults. Dexamethasone must be given either before or with the first dose of antibiotics and continued for 4 days. **Ⓐ**

The choice of empiric antibiotic coverage is guided by the most common pathogens for a patient's age group. In adolescents and adults < 50 years, most bacterial meningitis is caused by *S. pneumoniae* or *N. meningitides,* and a high-dose third-generation cephalosporin (ceftriaxone or cefotaxime) should be prescribed. **Ⓐ**

Adults > 50 years are also at risk for *L. monocytogenes,* and ampicillin should be added to the empiric regimen. **Ⓐ**

Vancomycin is added for empiric coverage of highly resistant *S. pneumoniae* while awaiting antibiotic sensitivities. **Ⓐ**

The antibiotic regimen should be adjusted when Gram stain and culture results are available.

Patients with recent head trauma or neurosurgery should be treated with ceftazidime or cefepime, instead of ceftriaxone or cefotaxime, for better coverage of aerobic Gram-negative rods. **Ⓐ**

Antibiotics should be given after blood cultures are obtained and lumbar puncture (LP) performed, *unless* a CT scan of the brain will be done prior to LP (*see* following Lab and Diagnostic Studies section). In this case, antibiotics should be given immediately after blood cultures. **Ⓑ**

Consultation with an infectious disease specialist is suggested for all patients with meningitis G to ensure that initial and long-term antibiotic choices are appropriate for these seriously ill patients.

Labs and Diagnostic Studies:

Blood cultures × 2 immediately, prior to antibiotics
CT scan of the brain
Cerebrospinal fluid (CSF) for cell count, differential, Gram stain, culture, protein, glucose, polymerase chain reaction (PCR) for enteroviruses

CBC with platelets, Chem 7, LFTs, prothrombin time (PT), partial thromboplastin time (PTT)

Blood cultures should always be obtained prior to administration of antibiotics and are positive in 50–70% of patients with bacterial meningitis. ❸

A CT scan of the brain prior to LP is recommended only for patients at significant risk for increased intracranial pressure and thus complications of LP. Risk factors identified in an observational study included:

- Age 60 and older
- Immunocompromised state
- Seizure in the week prior to presentation
- History of central nervous system (CNS) disease (i.e., stroke or infection)
- Decreased level of consciousness
- Abnormal neurologic exam

CT scan should be done prior to LP for patients with these risk factors and is not required for those without risk factors. ❹

LP with analysis of CSF should be performed in all patients with suspected meningitis. Opening pressure should be measured and is usually elevated in meningitis.

In untreated bacterial meningitis:

- CSF WBC is typically 1000–5000 cells, with a predominance of polymorphonuclear cells (PMNs)
- CSF glucose is < 40 mg/dL in 50–60% of patients
- CSF protein is elevated in > 90% of patients
- CSF Gram stain is positive in 60–90%
- CSF culture is positive in 70–85%

Even in patients who have not received antibiotics prior to LP, no test is perfect for diagnosing bacterial meningitis. Latex agglutination tests and PCR may be helpful in establishing a diagnosis when patients have been pretreated with antibiotics or when Gram stain and culture are negative; however, they should not be ordered routinely. ❸

Enteroviruses are the most common viral cause of meningitis. Enteroviral meningitis should be suspected in patients with lower CSF white counts with lymphocyte predominance and can be confirmed with PCR. Although there is no specific therapy, establishing the diagnosis can decrease the length of hospitalization and limit the use of antibiotics.

Discharge Planning:

Patients with bacterial meningitis typically require 2+ weeks of parenteral antibiotics, of which at least the initial 6 days should be given in the hospital. Completion of therapy with outpatient IV antibiotics can be considered for afebrile, clinically stable patients with no neurologic abnormalities, a safe and supportive home environment, and a clear plan for physician, nursing, and laboratory follow-up.

A peripherally inserted central catheter (PICC) line should be placed if outpatient therapy is planned.

The patient will require follow-up within 1 week of discharge with an infectious disease specialist or neurologist.

Special Considerations:

Infectious disease consultation is recommended for assistance with initial empiric and subsequent antibiotic choices. ❸

Patients with recent neurosurgery, head trauma, ventriculoperitoneal shunts, and immunosuppression may have other bacterial pathogens, including aerobic Gram-negative rods, coagulase-negative *Staphylococcus*, and others. Infectious disease consultation is especially appropriate for patients with these risk factors.

References

Hasbun R, Abrahams J, Jekel J, Ouagliarello VJ: Computed tomography of the head before lumbar puncture in adults with suspected meningitis. *N Engl J Med* 345:1727–1933, 2001.

Tunkel AR, Hartman BJ, Kaplan SL, et al: IDSA practice guidelines for the management of bacterial meningitis. *Clin Infect Dis* 39:1267–1284, 2004.

Osteomyelitis

Adults may develop osteomyelitis several ways: via hematogenous spread, via contiguous spread from an ulcer or soft tissue infection, or following surgery or trauma.

In adults, hematogenous osteomyelitis usually occurs in the setting of other risk factors, such as indwelling lines or catheters, dialysis, IDU, and recurrent urinary tract infection (UTI). It involves the vertebrae, pelvis, and sternoclavicular sites more commonly than long bones.

Patients with acute, hematogenously spread osteomyelitis are often systemically ill and are typically admitted for prompt evaluation and IV antibiotics.

Osteomyelitis in adults more commonly occurs in the setting of chronic ulcers due to diabetes or vascular disease or of decubiti. Many of these patients can be managed initially as outpatients.

Patients with suspected chronic osteomyelitis should be admitted if:

- Immediate surgical débridement or deep wound culture is needed
- Systemic signs of infection or sepsis is present
- There is associated soft tissue infection

- IV antibiotics are planned, and admission is necessary to coordinate ongoing care

These example orders are for a dialysis patient admitted with fever and pain in the sternoclavicular area, with suspected acute osteomyelitis.

A dmit to: Floor

D iagnosis: Osteomyelitis

C ondition: Stable

V ital Signs:
Routine

A llergies: Routine

A ctivity: Up as Tolerated, with Assistance

Pain from lower extremity or pelvic osteomyelitis may limit activity.

If vertebral osteomyelitis is suspected, evaluate the stability of the spine with plain films prior to allowing the patient to be up out of bed.

N ursing:
Routine. Call for temperature > 38.5°C, SBP < 100 mmHg, HR > 110 bpm

D iet: Regular

Check with surgical colleagues regarding potential need for NPO diet if preoperative.

IV Fluids: None Needed If Patient Able to Take PO

M edications:

Acetaminophen 650 mg PO q 6 hours prn pain or fever
Acetaminophen with codeine 1–2 tablets PO q 4 hours prn pain
Heparin 5000 units SQ q 8 hours

Antibiotic therapy is often withheld until positive blood cultures or bone cultures are obtained, unless contiguous soft tissue infection or sepsis is present. This allows identification of the causative organism to guide appropriate therapy. Inappropriate antibiotic therapy can lead to worse outcomes. **C**

If there is possible joint involvement, as in this patient with possible sternoclavicular osteomyelitis, an attempt to aspirate the joint should be made.

S. aureus is the most common organism causing acute osteomyelitis in adults, but aerobic Gram-negative rods cause 30% of cases.

Antibiotic choice should be guided by deep culture identification and sensitivities. There is very poor correlation between cultures of superficial wounds and deep cultures. **B**

Empiric antibiotic choices for patients with acute osteomyelitis would include: **C**

- Nafcillin, clindamycin, or cefazolin for suspected MSSA
- Vancomycin if there is concern for MRSA; for example in patients with IDU or recent exposure to a health care setting
- Levofloxacin if enteric aerobic Gram-negative rods are suspected, as in patients with recurrent UTIs, sickle cell disease, or IDU

The duration of antibiotic therapy is typically prolonged: 4–6 weeks. **C**

Labs and Diagnostic Studies:

Admit labs: CBC, erythrocyte sedimentation rate (ESR),
  C-reactive protein (CRP), chemistries, blood cultures × 2,
  UA and culture

Daily labs: CBC, chemistries if abnormal on admit,
  CRP × 3 days

Plain X-ray of the shoulder

There are several options for radiographic imaging in suspected osteomyelitis.

- Plain films are a rapid inexpensive first test and should be performed in all patients but can be negative in early acute osteomyelitis (i.e., the first several weeks).
- Three-phase technetium bone scan is more sensitive than plain film, but false positives may be caused by overlying ulceration or noninfectious etiologies of bone pain; for example, tumors, arthritis, or recent surgery. Bone scan is a good choice for evaluating suspected acute, uncomplicated long bone osteomyelitis.
- MRI is more sensitive than plain films and can help delineate soft tissue and bone involvement. MRI is the imaging study of choice in suspected diabetic foot osteomyelitis and vertebral osteomyelitis.
- CT evidence of osteomyelitis—for example, cortical destruction and soft tissue extension—can often be seen even when plain films are negative.

Positive blood cultures and clear radiographic evidence of osteomyelitis establish the diagnosis. However, this occurs in a minority of adult patients.

Bone biopsy, either CT guided or (less often) open, is usually pursued if blood cultures are not positive and imaging suggests osteomyelitis, both to establish the diagnosis and to obtain culture data to guide antibiotic therapy.

Discharge Planning:

Hematogenously spread osteomyelitis is typically treated with a prolonged course of IV antibiotics. **C**

Vertebral osteomyelitis necessitates 4–6 weeks of therapy. **B**

Contiguous osteomyelitis requires 4–6 weeks of therapy after débridement. **B**

A PICC line or other means of daily venous access should be arranged as soon as possible after blood cultures have become negative.

After initial IV therapy, a subspecialist may recommend switching to effective oral therapy for the duration of treatment.

A plan for postdischarge laboratory monitoring should be in place at the time of discharge from the hospital. For most antibiotics, postdischarge labs should include a CBC weekly for response to therapy and to monitor for drug toxicity plus an M7 weekly for drug toxicity (mostly renal).

Patient discharge education will include the signs and symptoms of worsening infection, the side effects of antimicrobials, and antibiotic administration and PICC care if IV therapy will be administered at home.

Special Considerations:

Infectious disease consultation is usually indicated to aid in diagnosis and antibiotic choices and to follow-up and manage outpatient antibiotics. **C**

Orthopedics consultation may be required for bone biopsy for culture and to assess for need for débridement of bone. **C**

Vascular surgery consultation should be obtained if osteomyelitis is secondary to diabetic or peripheral vascular ulcer. **C**

Infected hardware is increasingly associated with osteomyelitis.

When osteomyelitis occurs at the site of a foreign body, removal of that foreign body is optimal. However, in some cases, removal of hardware is not an option. When faced with this, adjust the duration of therapy in consultation with infectious disease and orthopedics. **Ⓑ**

References

Lew DP, Waldvogel FA: Osteomyelitis. *Lancet* 364:369–379, 2004.

pier.acponline.org/physicians/diseases/d592/d592.html.

Diabetic Foot Infection

Infected foot ulcers are a common cause for hospitalization of diabetics and precede almost all leg amputations in this population. Clinically, an infected foot ulcer is characterized by any two of the following findings:

- Purulent drainage
- Erythema
- Warmth
- Induration
- Pain or tenderness

Many patients can be managed as outpatients as long as timely multidisciplinary care is available. Admission to the hospital is indicated for:

- Systemic toxicity (fever, leukocytosis, tachycardia, hypotension, nausea and vomiting [N/V])
- Deep soft tissue infection (abscess, spread beneath superficial fascia) or cellulitis extending more than a few centimeters from the wound
- Critical limb ischemia
- Necrosis or gangrene

- Urgent diagnostic or therapeutic procedures
- Inability to manage at home
- Severe hyperglycemia or acidosis **C**

Admit to: Floor

Most patients with diabetic foot infections are stable enough for floor admission; rare patients have sepsis syndrome at admission and should be admitted to the ICU.

For the best outcome, a patient with a foot ulcer needs multidisciplinary care from a team usually including a primary care physician, diabetologist, wound specialist, podiatrist, footwear specialist, physical therapist, and often an infectious disease specialist and a vascular or orthopedic surgeon. **B**

Urgent surgical consultation is recommended for patients with critical ischemia or severe infections such as gas gangrene, necrotizing fasciitis, or sepsis syndrome. **B**

Diagnosis: Diabetic Foot Infection

Condition: Stable

Vital Signs:

Routine

Allergies: NKDA

Activity:

Strict non–weight-bearing right foot until orthotics consultation for special footwear

Off-loading the pressure from a foot wound is critical to healing. **B**

A variety of special shoes, orthotics, and splints may reduce pressure on the ulcer. These are usually fitted by a podiatrist or orthotist. Bedrest, crutches, and walkers alone are probably less effective than special footwear because it is difficult for patients to comply with non–weight-bearing, especially as outpatients.

Nursing:

Moist to dry gauze dressings to foot wound bid. Wound nurse consultation for further wound management recommendations

Check blood glucose qac and qhs

Moist to dry dressings are reasonable for initial wound management, but a moister environment is probably optimal for healing of most ulcers. Wound care nurses or specialists can recommend appropriate dressings for longer-term use. Wound specialists may also be able to débride any devitalized tissue to aid in healing.

Improved glycemic control may promote wound healing and decrease the risk of further infection.

Diet: Diabetic; No Concentrated Sugars

IV Fluids: None

Medications:

Piperacillin-tazobactam 3.375 g IV q 6 hours

NPH insulin 20 units SQ qAM and qhs

Regular insulin 8 units before breakfast and 10 units before dinner

Correction-dose insulin per low-dose algorithm
    (*see* **Diabetes Management, pp 275–280**)

Aspirin (ASA) 81 mg PO qd

Atorvastatin 20 mg PO qd

Nicotine patch 14 mg applied daily

The most common pathogens in diabetic foot infections are Gram-positive cocci, including *S. aureus*, beta-hemolytic strep, and coagulase-negative staphylococci. Mild diabetic foot infections can be treated with antibiotics aimed at

Gram positives, including dicloxacillin, cephalexin, amoxicillin-clavulanate, or TMP-SMX.

Most hospitalized patients, including those with more severe infections, ischemia, or chronic ulcers, should be empirically covered for Gram-negative and anaerobic pathogens as well. Antibiotic recommendations are primarily based on expert opinion and include:

- Piperacillin/tazobactam or ticarcillin/clavulanate
- Imipenem or another carbapenem
- Levofloxacin or ciprofloxacin, plus clindamycin
- Vancomycin plus ceftazidime for patients with or at high risk for MRSA

The duration of therapy for more severe infections is typically 2–3 weeks, longer if osteomyelitis is diagnosed. ❽

The empiric antibiotic regimen should be adjusted when culture results become available. Infectious disease consultation can be helpful in defining the optimal antibiotic regimen, both the choice of agent and duration of treatment.

Other evidence-based medical therapy is aimed at reducing the risk of progressive vascular disease in these high-risk patients: improved control of diabetes, lipid therapy, antiplatelet therapy, and smoking cessation.

Labs and Diagnostic Studies:

Admit: CBC, Chem 7, ESR, CRP, blood cultures
Plain films of the right foot
Vascular lab will perform bilateral ankle-brachial index (ABI) and arterial duplex if indicated
Deep wound culture will be performed after débridement by wound care specialist
Initial diagnostic studies should:

1. Establish the extent of infection and evaluate for osteomyelitis.

The extent of infection will determine the duration of antibiotic therapy and the need for surgical intervention. Plain films of the foot can demonstrate gas in the soft tissue, requiring urgent surgical débridement, or evidence of osteomyelitis, requiring at minimum a longer course of antibiotics. Many patients with ulcers have associated osteomyelitis, especially those with bone visible or palpable with a sterile probe. Plain films may be normal for the first 2–4 weeks, so normal films do not rule out the diagnosis. MRI is a more sensitive study for early osteomyelitis and can also evaluate for abscess or deep soft tissue infection if these are suspected clinically. MRI is preferred to nuclear isotope studies for evaluation of suspected osteomyelitis with nondiagnostic plain films. ❸

Elevated ESR and CRP increase the likelihood of osteomyelitis but are insensitive and nonspecific. Bone biopsy can establish both the diagnosis and the causative pathogen and susceptibilities in osteomyelitis.

2. Establish the pathogen.

Deep wound cultures and aspirates can identify the organism(s) causing infection and are preferred to superficial wound swabs, which typically grow multiple bacteria and are both nonspecific and insensitive for the causative organism. ❸

A deep wound culture should be obtained after débridement of necrotic superficial tissue. Purulent secretions can also be aspirated and sent for culture. If a deep culture has not been obtained prior to initial empiric therapy, one should definitely be done if the infection fails to improve.

3. Evaluate for ischemia contributing to ulceration.

If pulses are normal and the foot is warm, a vascular evaluation may not be necessary but should be performed if there is any suspicion for ischemia. An ABI of < 0.5 suggests that ischemia is contributing to ulceration. Diabetics may have calcified vessels, leading to falsely elevated

ABI, so an arterial duplex should be ordered if arterial insufficiency is still suspected with a normal or elevated ABI.

Discharge Planning:

Patients hospitalized with diabetic foot infections can be discharged when there has been an initial response and a definitive plan for therapy has been made. The plan of care must address:

- Follow-up physician, with a first visit for wound re-evaluation within 4–7 days
- Choice and estimated duration of antibiotics, which should be continued until the infection has resolved but not necessarily until the wound has healed **B**
- Off-loading pressure from the ulcer **A**
- Wound care, including repeat débridement if necessary **A**
- Glycemic control **C**

Patients with one diabetic ulcer are at very high risk for another. They should be evaluated for neuropathy and vascular disease and instructed in meticulous foot care, including daily foot inspection, moisturizers, nail care, and proper footwear. **C**

Patients should also be educated on diabetes management and modification of cardiovascular risk factors. **C**

Special Considerations:

A multidisciplinary approach is key to effective management of diabetic foot infections, both to preserve function and to avoid amputation. Because the consequences of inadequate therapy are high, specialists should be involved early if patients fail to respond to initial therapy. Surgical débridement or revascularization or adjustment of the antibiotic regimen could avert loss of the limb.

References

Cavanaugh PR, Lipsky BA, Bradbury AW, Botek G: Treatment for diabetic foot ulcers. *Lancet* 366:1725–1735, 2005.

Lipsky BA, Berendt AR, Deery HG: IDSA guidelines: Diagnosis and treatment of diabetic foot infections. *Clin Infect Dis* 34:885–910, 2004.

Pyelonephritis

The majority of pyelonephritis is uncomplicated, occurring in healthy patients without underlying abnormalities of the urinary tract. Most of these patients can be managed as outpatients with oral antibiotics. Patients with uncomplicated pyelonephritis should be admitted if they are unable to take oral fluids and medications or are toxic appearing, with high fever, tachycardia, or low BP.

Pyelonephritis is complicated when it occurs in the setting of a urinary catheter or stent or a functional or anatomic abnormality of the urinary system. The threshold for admission should be lower in patients with complicated UTI, and in immunosuppressed, recently hospitalized, or diabetic patients because these patients are more likely to have resistant organisms and be clinically sicker.

These orders are for a 31-year-old woman with acute pyelonephritis and vomiting.

Admit to: Floor

Most patients with pyelonephritis are stable enough to be admitted to the floor. If the patient has evidence of sepsis syndrome, admission to the ICU or a step-down unit should be considered. Diabetics are particularly prone to severe infection, including Gram-negative sepsis, and the condition of these patients may change quickly.

Diagnosis: Pyelonephritis

Condition: Stable

Vital Signs:

Routine

Allergies: Morphine

Activity: Ad Lib

Nursing:

Routine. Call for temperature > 38.5°C, SBP < 100 mmHg,
HR > 110 bpm

Patients with indwelling Foley catheters should have them
changed.

Diet: Clear Liquids Until Tolerating Oral Intake, then Advance Diet

Most patients admitted with pyelonephritis are nauseated
but can attempt to eat ASAP.

IVFluids: NS 250 mL/h × 2 Liters, then Call to Reassess

Aggressive volume replacement is necessary only if the patient
is hypovolemic from vomiting and decreased oral intake;
maintenance fluids should be prescribed if the patient is
euvolemic with inadequate oral intake.

Medications:

Ciprofloxacin 400 mg IV q 12 hours
Phenergan 12.5–25 mg IV q 6 hours prn nausea

Initial empiric therapy of uncomplicated pyelonephritis should cover enteric Gram-negative pathogens, which are the most common cause. IV fluoroquinolones are commonly prescribed; ceftriaxone is an alternative, although it does not cover enterococci and should not be used if Gram-positive cocci are seen on Gram stain. **Ⓐ**

If Gram-positive cocci are seen on Gram stain in uncomplicated pyelonephritis, IV ampicillin-sulbactam should be prescribed to cover enterococcus. **Ⓐ**

Choose a broader-spectrum antibiotic, such as piperacillin/tazobactam or a carbapenem, if *Pseudomonas* or other resistant Gram-negatives are suspected in cases of complicated UTI. Some authorities also suggest empiric coverage of staphylococci, including MRSA, in complicated UTI. **Ⓒ**

In pregnancy, IV ceftriaxone or ampicillin-gentamicin should be used as initial therapy because quinolones are contraindicated.

When vomiting resolves, select an oral antibiotic based on culture and sensitivies. Pathogen susceptibility to fluoroquinolones is still very high. TMP-SMX resistance is 20% in some areas. Nitrofurantoin is a reasonable alternative in women with allergy or resistance to first-line antibacterials, but it is not as effective in men.

Labs and Diagnostic Studies:

UA, Gram stain and culture
CBC, Chem 7
CBC: WBC typically elevated. M7: an elevated creatinine suggests obstruction; investigate further with renal ultrasound to look for kidney stones and abscess

Pyuria is found in most patients with pyelonephritis. Gram-negative organisms are often visible on microscopic exam. Urine culture is mandatory in inpatients to determine antibiotic susceptibility. Whenever possible, obtain culture prior to initial antibiotic therapy. **Ⓒ**

Blood cultures are positive in a minority of patients with uncomplicated pyelonephritis but should be done in most patients who are admitted, including those with complicated pyelonephritis. **C**

WBC is typically elevated in pyelonephritis and falls with appropriate therapy. Elevated serum creatinine, hematuria, or renal colic suggest urinary obstruction. In such cases, an ultrasound should be performed on admission because infection will not improve unless the obstruction is resolved. **B**

In diabetics, some experts recommend imaging the kidneys at admission, with plain films or ultrasound, to exclude the diagnosis of emphysematous pyelonephritis, in which gas-forming organisms form visible air in the renal parenchyma. **C**

If at 48–72 hours after admission the patient remains febrile and WBC has not improved, or if overall there has been no clinical improvement, obtain CT scan of the kidneys to rule out renal abscess or emphysematous pyelonephritis. **B**

D ischarge Planning:

Patients may be discharged when they are able to take oral nutrition and medication and have defervesced.

Treat with 10–14 days of antibiotics and perform follow-up urine culture to document infection clearance.

S pecial Considerations:

Nearly all patients improve within 24–48 hours unless there is a complicating factor such as renal abscess or antibiotic resistance.

In pregnancy, complications of severe pyelonephritis include preterm labor and delivery; the patient's obstetrician should be consulted early.

References

Hooton TM: The current management strategies for community-acquired UTI. *Infect Dis Clin North Am* 17:303–332, 2003.

Stamm WE, Hooton TM: Management of UTI in adults. *N Engl J Med* 329:1328–1334, 1993.

Acute Arthritis

Acute arthritis may be due to infection, crystal arthritis, or other rheumatologic disease. If the cause is rheumatologic, admission is usually indicated only if the patient is unable to ambulate or has other systemic manifestations requiring inpatient treatment. Patients with acute bacterial arthritis should be admitted to the hospital for rapid orthopedic consultation, drainage of the affected joint, and initiation of IV antibiotic therapy because significant joint destruction and permanent dysfunction may result from any delay in treatment.

A dmit to: Floor

Patients with acute arthritis can be managed on the floor unless they have hypotension or other evidence of sepsis syndrome. If endocarditis with secondary seeding of the joint is suspected, the patient should be placed on telemetry.

D iagnosis: Acute Arthritis

C ondition: Serious

Condition may range from stable to critical, depending on cause and presentation.

Patients with acute bacterial arthritis may be seriously ill with systemic signs of sepsis. Acute arthritis may be the initial manifestation of bacterial endocarditis, particularly in patients with a history of IDU.

V ital Signs:

Routine

Be vigilant for vital signs that suggest impending sepsis (tachycardia, hypotension, hypothermia, or hyperthermia). If these develop, increase frequency of vital signs.

A llergies: Routine

A ctivity: As Tolerated

Weight bearing should be avoided on joints immobilized by septic arthritis, but range of motion (ROM) as tolerated should be provided by physical therapy.

N ursing:

Elevate the affected extremity while supine

Acute arthritis is often accompanied by edema of the associated extremity, which may be aided by elevation above the level of the heart.

D iet: Regular

The patient should be made NPO if it is suspected he or she will need surgical washout.

IV Fluids: Heplock

Maintenance IV fluids are not necessary if the patient is able to eat and drink.

Medications:

Tylenol 650 mg PO q 4–6 hours prn, ibuprofen 600 mg PO q
   6 hours prn, oxycodone 5–10 mg PO q 4 hours prn,
   docusate 250 mg PO bid
Empiric antibiotics should not be administered before obtaining
   synovial fluid for Gram stain and culture.
   Suggested empiric regimens:

- Adult with monoarticular arthritis, at risk for sexually transmitted disease (STD): Ceftriaxone 1 g IV qd
- Adult with monoarticular arthritis, not at risk for STD: Nafcillin 2 g IV q 4 hours *plus* ceftriaxone 1 g IV qd. If the patient has a history of IDU or other risk factors for MRSA (recent incarceration or hospitalization), add vancomycin 1 g IV q 12 hours while awaiting cultures
- Adult with polyarticular arthritis: Ceftriaxone 1 g IV qd

If intracellular crystals are present in synovial fluid, begin therapy for crystal arthritis. Options are NSAIDs (typically indomethacin), colchicine, and oral or intraarticular steroids. Allopurinol should not be started in the setting of acute gout because it will exacerbate symptoms.

Labs and Diagnostic Studies:

Synovial fluid for cell count and differential, crystal examination,
   Gram stain and culture
CBC with differential, Chem 7, blood cultures × 2, ESR, CRP,
   uric acid
   Synovial fluid analysis is critical in the evaluation of acute arthritis. Only 1–2 mL of fluid is necessary for complete analysis.
   Synovial fluid WBC $> 50,000/mm^3$ suggests bacterial infection, which is confirmed by positive Gram stain or culture. Septic arthritis causes rapid joint destruction and loss of

function, so early diagnosis and orthopedic consultation is crucial in management, especially for weight-bearing joints.

The presence of intracellular crystals confirms the diagnosis of gout or pseudogout. Serum uric acid may be normal in acute gout, but a very elevated level suggests gout as the diagnosis.

Gonorrhea can also cause acute arthritis. If the patient is at risk for STD, cervical, urethral, pharyngeal, and/or rectal swabs should be sent for culture.

Discharge Planning:

Prior to discharge, signs of inflammation should be improving and pain should be controlled.

Physical therapy should be consulted early for ROM and postdischarge exercise plan.

Septic arthritis is typically treated with a prolonged course of IV antibiotics. A PICC line should be considered, and if the antibiotics are to be administered at home, home infusion service and infectious disease follow-up arranged.

Special Considerations:

Septic arthritis can lead to rapid destruction of a joint and permanent disability. All authorities agree on the need for prompt drainage of affected joints, but there is no consensus and limited data on whether drainage should be operative (usually arthroscopic) or via daily arthrocentesis. Prompt orthopedic or rheumatology consultation is recommended if septic arthritis is suspected.

References

Baker DG, Schmacher HR: Acute monoarthritis. *N Engl J Med* 329:1013–1020, 1993.

Cibere J: Rheumatology: 4. Acute monoarthritis. *CMAJ* 162:1577–1583, 2000.

Gilbert D, Moellering RC, Eliopoulos GM, Sancle M: *The Sanford Guide to Antimicrobial Therapy 2004*, ed 34. Septic Arthritis. Hyde Park, VT, Antimicrobial Therapy Inc., 2004.

Goldenberg DL: Septic arthritis. *Lancet* 351:197–202, 1998.

Kerr LD: Inflammatory arthritis in the elderly. *Mt Sinai J Med* 70:23–26, 2003.

Li SF, Henderson J, Dickman E, et al: Laboratory tests in adults with monoarticular arthritis: can they rule out a septic joint? *Acad Emerg Med* 11:276–280, 2004.

Manadam AM, Block JA: Daily needle aspiration versus surgical lavage for the treatment of bacterial septic arthritis in adults. *Am J Ther* 11:412–415, 2004.

Nade S: Septic arthritis. *Best Pract Res Clin Rheum* 17:183–200, 2003.

Pinals RS: Polyarthritis and fever. *N Engl J Med* 330:769–774, 1994.

Shirtliff ME, Mader JT: Acute septic arthritis. *Clin Microbiol Rev* 15:527–544, 2002.

Severe Sepsis and Septic Shock

Sepsis is the systemic response to a severe infection. A consensus panel has developed definitions for sepsis across a continuum of severity:

Systemic inflammatory response syndrome (SIRS) may occur with infection or other severe insults and is defined as any two of:

- Temperature $> 38°C$ or $< 36°C$
- HR > 90 bpm
- RR > 20 breaths/min or $PaCO_2 < 32$ mmHg
- WBC $> 12,000/mm^3$ or $< 4000/mm^3$, or 10% bands

Sepsis: SIRS with documented infection

Severe sepsis: Sepsis with hypotension, evidence of hypoperfusion, or organ dysfunction

Septic shock: Sepsis with hypotension despite fluid resuscitation and end-organ evidence of hypoperfusion, such as decreased urine output (UO) or altered mental status

These orders apply to patients with severe sepsis and septic shock; that is, patients with hypotension, organ dysfunction, or evidence of hypoperfusion.

A dmit to: ICU

Patients with severe sepsis or septic shock should be admitted to the ICU for close monitoring and treatment. ●

D iagnosis: Severe Sepsis and Septic Shock

C ondition: Critical

Severe sepsis and septic shock have a high mortality (15–40%). Sepsis is the leading noncardiac cause of death in American ICUs.

V ital Signs:

Every 15 minutes × 4, then hourly if initially stable

Call for BP < 90/60 mmHg, HR > 120 bpm, worsening oxygenation, UO < 30 mL/h

Patients with severe sepsis and septic shock should have vital signs performed at least every hour, more frequently in the first hours of admission. A BP cuff may be inaccurate in patients with sepsis. If BP is labile or persistently low, consider an arterial line for monitoring after initial evaluation and fluid resuscitation are underway.

A llergies: Routine

A ctivity: Bedrest

N ursing:

Foley catheter
Strict I/Os
Daily weight
Neurologic checks q 2 hours—call for worsening neurologic status

Fluid resuscitation is crucial to the management of sepsis, but intake is typically much higher than UO in the first 24–48 hours due to vasodilation and capillary leak.

Mental status changes may indicate progression to septic shock, and nursing staff should be instructed to call if the patient's mental status worsens.

D iet: NPO

Patients with severe sepsis are critically ill and usually unable to eat. Patients with confusion or respiratory compromise potentially requiring intubation should not eat, even if they are able to do so, because of the risk of aspiration pneumonia.

IV Fluids: NS 500 mL Every 30 Minutes Until Central Venous Pressure (CVP) > 8 mmHg, then Continue NS at 150 mL/h

Fluid resuscitation should begin as soon as severe sepsis is recognized in the emergency room. Adequate early resuscitation can support tissue perfusion, and in a trial of early goal-directed therapy of severe sepsis, it reduced mortality. **Ⓐ**

At least two large-bore IV lines should be placed to allow adequate fluid resuscitation. It may be difficult to obtain adequate peripheral IV access in patients with sepsis and hypoperfusion—in this case, a large-bore central line (Cordis) can be placed.

The patient's volume status should be reassessed frequently to ensure adequate resuscitation but to avoid iatrogenic pulmonary edema. CVP may be measured with a central venous catheter, or the physician may examine the jugular venous pressure if a central line has not been placed. **Ⓒ**

Medications:

Vancomycin 1 g IV q 12 hours
Imipenem 500 mg IV q 6 hours
Insulin drip per ICU protocol, to maintain blood glucose 80–150 mg/dL
Ranitidine 150 mg IV qd
Hydrocortisone 50 mg IV q 6 hours
Heparin 5000 units SQ q 8 hours

The choice of empiric antibiotics depends on the probable source of infection, recent antibiotic use, and local resistance patterns and should be individualized for each patient. Consider early infectious disease consultation for assistance with antibiotic choices.

In general, however, initial therapy should be very broad because inadequate antibiotic coverage is associated with increased mortality in sepsis. **Ⓑ**

MRSA is increasingly recognized as a cause of severe infection and sepsis, even in community patients. If the source of severe sepsis/septic shock is not clear, the initial regimen should cover MRSA (usually with vancomycin, although daptomycin is an alternative) until it has been excluded. **Ⓒ**

Other organisms should also be covered broadly until the source of infection is clear. A carbapenem or third- or fourth-generation cephalosporin may be used for initial coverage. If a patient has recently been treated with an antibiotic, use an alternate antibiotic class. If *Pseudomonas* sepsis is strongly suspected, some experts would recommend double coverage, adding a quinolone, antipseudomonal aminoglycoside, or piperacillin/tazobactam. Up-to-date antibiotic guidelines may be found in Gilbert, et al, 2005 (updated yearly). **B**

After initial stabilization, glucose control is a priority. Even nondiabetic patients are likely to be hyperglycemic under the stress of sepsis. Tight glycemic control (80–110 mg/dL) in critically ill postoperative patients has been shown to increase survival and decrease infection. Randomized trials of medical ICU patients have not been published, but most experts recommend controlling glucose in patients with sepsis, with a target glucose of 80–150 mg/dL. An insulin infusion protocol is the safest and most effective way of accomplishing this. **C**

Stress ulcer prophylaxis with ranitidine should be instituted. **A**

Randomized trials of patients with severe septic shock requiring vasopressors have shown improved outcomes with IV corticosteroids. A cosyntropin stimulation test should be done (*see* following Labs and Diagnostic Studies section) to assess for relative adrenal insufficiency, but steroids should be started in patients with hypotension that has not resolved with fluids while waiting for results. If results are normal, hydrocortisone may be stopped. **A**

Deep vein thrombosis (DVT) prophylaxis should be prescribed for all ICU patients. Options include unfractionated heparin, low-molecular-weight heparin, or if heparin is contraindicated, sequential compression devices (SCDs). **A**

Recombinant activated protein C (Xigris) should be considered if a patient is at high risk of death based on Acute Physiology and Chronic Health Evaluation (APACHE) II score, multiple organ failure, or acute respiratory distress syndrome (ARDS). **Ⓐ**

Because recombinant activated protein C increases the risk of bleeding, this drug is absolutely contraindicated in patients with active bleeding, recent hemorrhagic stroke, recent neurosurgery, trauma, intracranial mass lesion, or epidural catheter. If you are considering administering activated protein C, consultation with an experienced critical care or infectious disease specialist is recommended. **Ⓒ**

L abs and Diagnostic Studies:

On admission: Blood cultures × 3, UA and culture, CBC with differential and platelet count, Chem 7, calcium, magnesium, LFTs, amylase, PT, PTT, thrombin time, fibrinogen level, serum lactate level, arterial blood gas, ECG, CXR

Perform cosyntropin stimulation test:

1. Draw serum cortisol
2. Give cosyntropin 250 μg IV
3. Redraw serum cortisol 30 and 60 minutes later

Daily: CBC with differential, Chem 7, calcium, magnesium, PT, PTT

Initial lab and diagnostic studies are aimed at:

1. Identifying the source of sepsis. Control of the source is critical to successful management of severe sepsis
2. Establishing the severity of illness

Blood cultures and urine culture should be done on all patients as soon after presentation as possible and before the administration of antibiotics (which should occur quickly). **Ⓑ**

A CXR should also be done in all patients because sepsis due to pneumonia may present with a paucity of pulmonary symptoms. Severe pancreatitis may mimic sepsis syndrome, even in the absence of infected tissue, so a serum amylase should be done if another source of sepsis is not obvious. **C**

Elevated serum lactate level indicates end-organ hypoperfusion. Abnormal PT, PTT, thrombin time, fibrinogen, and platelets may indicate the patient is developing disseminated intravascular coagulation as a complication of sepsis. **C**

Further diagnostic studies to identify the source of sepsis are guided by the initial evaluation. It is critically important that any identified source of sepsis is controlled as quickly as possible (e.g., abscess drainage, débridement of infected tissue, or removal of an infected line or device). **C**

The cosyntropin stimulation test identifies patients with septic shock and relative adrenal insufficiency who will benefit from continued treatment with IV corticosteroids. **A**

Discharge Planning:

Patients with severe sepsis may not survive to discharge from the ICU. Daily communication between the ICU care team and the patient's family can help define the goals of care and ensure decisions are made in the patient's best interest.

Special Considerations:

If the patient develops respiratory failure requiring intubation, a lung-protective ventilation strategy should be instituted using tidal volumes of 6 mL/kg/min. **A**

Ventilated patients should be laid in the semirecumbent position (at 45 degrees) to reduce the risk of ventilator-associated pneumonia. **A**

References

Dellinger RP, Carlet JM, Masur H, et al: Surviving Sepsis Campaign guidelines for management of severe sepsis and septic shock. *Crit Care Med* 32:858–873, 2004.

Gilbert D, Moellering RC, Eliopoulos GM, Sande M: *The Sanford Guide to Antimicrobial Therapy 2005*. Hyde Park, VT, Antimicrobial Therapy, Inc., 2005.

Pulmonary Tuberculosis

Although the incidence of pulmonary TB is declining, multidrug-resistant TB and nosocomial transmission are still problematic. TB should be suspected and respiratory isolation and diagnostic testing instituted for any patient with pulmonary infiltrates and:

- Cavitation
- Miliary pattern
- Upper lobe predominance
- More than 1 month of cough, fever, sweats, malaise, weakness, or significant weight loss

The index of suspicion for TB should be even higher for patients who are immunosuppressed, are foreign born, or have a history of incarceration.

Those with HIV and CD4 count < 200 cells can have TB without typical findings on CXR.

Many patients can be evaluated as outpatients; those with severe symptoms and those whose social situation increases risk of transmission (i.e., homelessness, incarceration) are typically admitted.

Admit to: Floor; Negative Pressure Room and Airborne Isolation Precautions

Prompt isolation is essential to prevent nosocomial transmission of TB. Patients with suspected TB should be admitted to a room with negative pressure ventilation, and all health care personnel entering the patient's room should use a fit-tested N95 respirator or powered air purifying respirator (PAPR).

Patients should remain in isolation until:

- Active TB is excluded *or*
- Discharge from the hospital *or*
- Therapy has been initiated and the patient is felt to be no longer infectious

Diagnosis: Pulmonary Tuberculosis

Condition: Stable

Vital Signs:

Routine

Vital signs (temperature, BP, HR, and RR, including oxygen saturation) on admission, then every shift.

Allergies: NKDA

Activity: Encourage Activity as Tolerated, In the Room

Patients with suspected TB should not travel outside of their rooms except for necessary diagnostic tests and procedures, to avoid placing other patients and health care workers at unnecessary risk.

Nursing:

Weigh patient on admission

Weight is necessary for appropriate drug dosing.

D iet: Regular

If the patient is unable to cough up any sputum and requires sputum induction, he or she should be NPO after midnight prior to induction.

IV Fluids: None

No IV fluids are necessary if the patient is able to eat and is not volume depleted.

M edications:

Tylenol 325–650 mg orally q 4–6 hours as needed for fever; not to exceed 4 g in 24 hours

The definitive diagnosis of TB is based on culture, which may take weeks, but the diagnosis may be strongly suspected based on clinical presentation or positive sputum acid-fast bacilli (AFB) smears. The timing of initiation of therapy depends on the severity of illness and how strongly TB is suspected. Consultation with infectious disease or the local public health department may be helpful. The choice of initial therapy should be based on local drug-resistance patterns. ❸

For areas with local prevalence of isoniazid resistance > 4% (found in 33 states in 1997), the first-line regimen is:

- Isoniazid 5 mg/kg PO qd (not to exceed 300 mg PO qd) *and*
- Pyridoxine 25–50 mg PO qd *and*
- Rifampin 10 mg/kg PO qd (not to exceed 600 mg PO qd) *and*
- Pyrazinamide 25 mg/kg PO qd *and*
- Ethambutol 15–25 mg/kg PO qd

Symptomatic hepatotoxicity is estimated to occur in 1–3 per 1000 persons treated with isoniazid. Because the most important cofactor for the development of hepatotoxicity is alcohol consumption, patients should be advised to avoid alcohol while on the drug. Isoniazid should not be given if a symptomatic patient's serum transaminase level is greater than three times the upper limit of normal or if an asymptomatic patient's serum transaminase level is greater than five times the upper limit of normal.

Pyridoxine is given concurrently with isoniazid to prevent neuropathy.

Rifampin can also cause hepatotoxicity and should not be given if a symptomatic patient's serum transaminase level is greater than three times the upper limit of normal or if an asymptomatic patient's serum transaminase level is greater than five times the upper limit of normal.

If the local prevalence of resistance to isoniazid is ≥ 4%, a fourth agent, such as ethambutol, should be added. In 1997 in 33 states, 14% of isolates were resistant to isoniazid; therefore the recommended initial regimen is four-drug therapy.

Duration of treatment for drug-susceptible TB is at least 6 months. The public health department should be involved in follow-up and decisions on duration of therapy for patients with documented TB.

Labs and Diagnostic Studies:

CBC with differential, Chem 7, LFTs
Obtain sputum samples for AFB smear and culture every day for 3 days (at least 8 hours between samples obtained)
PA and lateral CXR
Place purified protein derivative (PPD) unless current PPD status known
HIV serology after consent

CBC with differential and kidney and liver function should be checked prior to initiation of any therapy for TB.

Sputum samples for AFB smear and culture should be obtained each day for the first 3 days of hospitalization, with at least 8 hours between samples. The sensitivity of smears is 50–70%, and of culture, 80–85%. **ⓐ**

Sputum samples are best obtained early in the morning.

Culture is required for all patients for definitive diagnosis and susceptibility testing. Cultures should be maintained for at least 6 weeks.

If the first sputum result is smear positive, discontinue further sputum collection.

If patient cannot produce expectorated sputum, sputum should be induced by administration of nebulized saline (usually by respiratory therapy). The yield from a single induced sputum was equivalent to bronchoscopy in one study. **ⓑ**

If induced sputum cannot be obtained and clinical suspicion for TB remains, consult pulmonary to perform bronchoscopy and obtain bronchoalveolar lavage (BAL) specimen for AFB smear and culture. **ⓑ**

All patients diagnosed with pulmonary TB should be strongly encouraged to undergo HIV testing within 2 months of TB diagnosis.

Although most patients with pulmonary TB have an abnormal CXR, the sensitivity and specificity of any given finding is low, particularly in patients who are immunocompromised. Chest CT is more sensitive in identifying early active disease. No CXR or CT finding can replace sputum analysis for diagnosis of pulmonary TB.

Skin testing is neither sensitive nor specific for a diagnosis of TB but can be helpful in initial clinical decision making. It is recommended in all persons at high risk for latent TB, including patients with HIV infection, IDU, homelessness, incarceration, or contact with any person with active pulmonary TB.

Discharge Planning:

Pulmonary TB is a reportable condition in most states, and the public health department should be notified of confirmed diagnoses. The public health department can also help in planning for discharge.

Directly observed therapy (DOT) is highly recommended to help ensure higher completion rates, prevent the emergence of drug-resistant TB, and enhance TB control. DOT may be available through the local public health agency.

The public health department can often also help with follow-up, adjustment of medication regimens, surveillance for development of toxicity, drug-resistant strains, and failure of therapy.

Patients with three negative smears—surrogate for infectiousness—are usually considered to be noninfectious and isolation can be discontinued. For patients with sputum samples positive for AFB, continue isolation for a minimum of 2 weeks of therapy. A longer period of isolation may be recommended for patients with HIV and those with multidrug–resistant TB.

Patients may be discharged to home before their sputum smears become negative but should not be discharged to a skilled nursing facility (SNF), jail, a shelter, or the street while still infectious.

Discharge education should include a careful review of medications and side effects, including instructions to avoid alcohol and to stop medications and come in for follow-up immediately if signs of hepatotoxicity (nausea, right upper quadrant [RUQ] pain, or jaundice) occur.

Special Considerations:

Prompt consultation with an infectious disease specialist and/or the local public health department is recommended in cases of suspected multidrug-resistant TB.

References

Al Zahrani K, Al Jahdali H, Poirier L, et al: Accuracy and utility of commercially available amplification and serologic tests for the diagnosis of minimal pulmonary tuberculosis. *Am J Respir Crit Care Med* 162:1323–1329, 2000.

Anderson C, Inhaber N, Menzies D: Comparison of sputum induction with fiber-optic bronchoscopy in the diagnosis of tuberculosis. *Am J Respir Crit Care Med* 152:1570–1574, 1995.

Blumberg HM, Leonard MK, Jasmer RM, et al: Update on the treatment of tuberculosis and latent tuberculosis infection. *JAMA* 293:2776–2784, 2005.

Kunimoto D, Long R: Tuberculosis: Still overlooked as a cause of community-acquired pneumonia—how not to miss it. *Respir Care Clin North Am* 11:25–34, 2005.

Merrick ST, Sepkowitz KA, Walsh J, et al: Comparison of induced versus expectorated sputum for diagnosis of pulmonary tuberculosis by acid-fast smear. *Am J Infect Control* 25:463–466, 1997.

Nelson SM, Duke MA, Cartwright CP, et al: Value of examining multiple sputum specimens in the diagnosis of pulmonary tuberculosis. *J Clin Microbiol* 36:467–469, 1998.

Central Line Infection

Admission with central line infection is increasingly common as more outpatients have indwelling lines such as dialysis catheters, Hickman catheters, Portacaths, and PICCs.

Patients with indwelling catheters should be evaluated for line infection any time they develop fever.

Coagulase-negative staphylococci are the most common microbiologic cause, and patients infected with these organisms often present with fever alone.

However, more virulent organisms such as *S. aureus,* *Candida albicans,* and Gram-negative rods can also cause line infections, and patients infected with these organisms can be substantially sicker.

Clinically stable patients with fever but no evidence of sepsis and a normal examination of the line may have blood cultures drawn as outpatients, if very close follow-up is available.

Patients with any evidence of sepsis, infection of the tunnel or exit site, immunosuppression, or inadequate social situation or follow-up should be admitted for further evaluation and management.

Initial management of suspected line infections requires both treatment with an appropriate antibiotic and a decision to remove or attempt to salvage the line, which should usually be made within the first 24–48 hours.

These orders are for a dialysis patient admitted with fever and erythema at the exit site of her dialysis catheter.

A dmit to: Floor

Most patients with line infection are stable enough to be admitted to the floor. However, infection with virulent organisms may lead to sepsis syndrome, requiring admission to an ICU or step-down unit. Patients with sepsis syndrome and suspected line infection should have the line removed immediately. *See* Severe Sepsis and Septic Shock, pp 182–189 for further recommendations for management of sepsis. **C**

Patients with a history of MRSA infection should be placed in contact isolation until MRSA is ruled out.

D iagnosis: Central Line Infection

C ondition: Serious

Patients with line infection are often bacteremic and can decompensate quickly.

V ital Signs:

Every 2 hours × 2, then if stable, per routine. Call for HR > 110 bpm, SBP < 100 mmHg, RR > 24 breaths/minute, decreased UO
Vital sign changes, including tachypnea and tachycardia, can be early indicators of severe sepsis, as can decreased UO. ❽

A llergies: Routine

A ctivity: Activity as Tolerated

N ursing:

Daily weights, strict I/Os, dressing change to line per routine
Daily weights and I/Os can be discontinued if the patient does not develop evidence of sepsis in the first 24–48 hours.

D iet: Renal

Consider making patients with lines that must be removed in the operating room (e.g., Portacaths) NPO until the time of removal is determined.

Dialysis patients should have a renal diet. If the dialysis catheter will need to be removed until blood cultures clear on antibiotics, consider ordering a more strict fluid-restriction/low-potassium diet, because dialysis will need to be delayed until the catheter is replaced.

IV Fluids: Place a Peripheral IV and Heplock

IV fluids should be ordered only if needed; avoid unnecessary fluids and potassium in patients with renal failure.

M edications:

Vancomycin 1 g IV now
Tylenol 325–650 mg PO q 6 hours prn pain/fever
Continue outpatient medications

Empiric antibiotics must be tailored to the individual patient but should generally provide excellent Gram-positive coverage, including MRSA for patients at risk. Vancomycin is commonly prescribed as empiric therapy for line infections, especially in dialysis patients, for whom the dosing interval is as long as 5–7 days. **❸**

If the patient has had a recent prior line infection, ensure the initial antibiotic regimen covers that pathogen. **❸**

Patients with sepsis syndrome and those with neutropenia should receive broader therapy while awaiting culture results—*see* Severe Sepsis and Septic Shock, pp 182–189; Febrile Neutropenia, pp 137–142.

Antibiotics should be adjusted when culture and sensitivity results are available, using other antibiotics as appropriate, to avoid overuse of and resistance to vancomycin. **❸**

Infectious disease consultation may be helpful in choosing the most appropriate antibiotic and duration of therapy. **❸**

Antibiotic lock therapy (instillation of antibiotic solution in each port of the catheter) can improve the rate of salvage of permanent catheters infected with staphylococci. **❸**

Labs and Diagnostic Studies:

On admission: Blood cultures—two (one from line, one from peripheral site), *before* antibiotics are administered
CBC with differential, Chem 7, UA, urine culture; CXR, PA and lateral
Daily CBC, repeat blood cultures daily until negative

Blood cultures should be obtained from the line and from a peripheral site prior to administration of antibiotics, which can decrease the sensitivity of cultures. **❹**

If it is not known whether the line is the source of bacteremia, quantitative cultures of blood drawn peripherally should be compared with blood drawn through the line. If the bacterial colony count of blood drawn from the line is higher, the line is the likely source of bacteremia. **❹**

Blood cultures should be performed daily until they are sterile to document response to therapy and to determine when a new line can be placed. Blood cultures that remain positive for more than 2 days after removal of an infected line should suggest a complicating factor such as suppurative thrombophlebitis or endocarditis. **C**

Consider adding fungal blood cultures if the patient is immunosuppressed. *Candida* is more common in patients on total parenteral nutrition (TPN) but will usually grow from standard blood cultures. **C**

If the patient's line is removed, the tip should be sent under sterile conditions for quantitative culture. This can be done with a sterile scissors and collection container. **A**

If the patient's blood cultures are positive for *S. aureus,* a transesophageal echocardiogram can help rule out secondary endocarditis to determine the appropriate duration of therapy. **A**

D ischarge Planning:

Length of stay will depend on the severity of infection and whether a new line will be required or salvage will be attempted. Most patients will continue to need central venous access and will typically require a course of IV antibiotics. Blood cultures should be clear for at least 48 hours prior to placement of a new line. **B**

Patients should be educated on appropriate care of the line prior to discharge. **C**

S pecial Considerations:

Initial management of suspected line infections requires both appropriate antibiotic therapy and a decision to remove or attempt to salvage the line. The line should be removed at admission if the patient has sepsis syndrome, if it is no longer necessary, or if the line tunnel or pocket is infected based on exam. ●

An attempt to salvage a line also depends on the necessity of the line, the difficulty of replacing it, and the isolated organism. Coagulase-negative *Staphylococcus* infections are often curable with systemic and antibiotic lock therapy, whereas other organisms typically require removal of the line for cure. Infectious disease consultation may be helpful.

References

Allon M: Dialysis catheter-related bacteremia: Prophylaxis and treatment. *Am J Kidney Dis* 44:779–791, 2004.

Mermel LA, Farr BM, Shevetz RJ, et al: IDSA guidelines for the management of central venous catheter infections. *Clin Infect Dis* 32:1249–1272, 2001.

Safdar N, Fine JP, Maki DG, et al: Meta-analysis: methods for diagnosing intravascular device–related bloodstream infection. *Ann Intern Med* 142:451–466, 2005.

Fever of Unknown Origin

Fever of unknown origin (FUO) is defined as:

- A temperature > 38.3°C on several occasions
- Lasting longer than 3 weeks
- Despite at least 1 week of evaluation, classically in the hospital but now more often in the clinic

Patients with FUO may be admitted to facilitate evaluation or because they appear toxic or have another indication for hospitalization.

Three major categories of disease cause FUO:

- Infection
- Malignancy

- Inflammatory diseases

The prognosis depends on the ultimate diagnosis. About 30% of patients with FUO never have a cause defined; the prognosis for these patients is good.

A dmit to: Floor

Most patients with FUO are stable enough to be admitted to the floor. Patients with evidence of sepsis should be managed differently (*see* Severe Sepsis and Septic Shock, pp 182–189).

D iagnosis: FUO

C ondition: Stable

The prognosis depends on the ultimate diagnosis.

V ital Signs:

Vital signs, including temperature q 4 hours

The temperature should be monitored frequently to document that fever is in fact still present.

A llergies: NKDA

A ctivity: Ad Lib

N ursing:

Call for temperature > 38°C

Reassessment when the patient is febrile may offer clues in some cases. Patients with Still's disease may have a transitory rash, and blood cultures at the time of fever may be more likely to be positive.

D iet: General

Remember to consider planned diagnostic testing and whether NPO status is required.

IV Fluids: None

M edications:

No acetaminophen, ibuprofen, or aspirin

Because drugs can be a cause of fever, patients admitted with FUO should receive only medications that are absolutely necessary. If fever has not resolved within 72 hours of stopping a drug, it is not likely to be the cause. ©

Antipyretics should be withheld, at least initially, so that true fever can be documented.

Unless a patient has sepsis syndrome or severe immunocompromise (especially neutropenia), antibiotics should generally not be prescribed for FUO because empiric antibiotics are more likely to cloud the picture than lead to a cure. ©

L abs and Diagnostic Studies:

CBC with differential and smear evaluation, Chem 7, LFTs, UA and culture, blood cultures × 3, antinuclear antibody (ANA), rheumatoid factor, HIV serology, cytomegalovirus (CMV) IgM antibody, Monospot, PA and lateral CXR

These initial labs have been recommended as the minimal diagnostic work-up that must be done for a fever to quality as FUO. ©

CBC with differential and an evaluation of the peripheral smear by a hematopathologist can lead to a diagnosis of hematologic malignancy or an autoimmune cause of fever. At least three sets of blood cultures should be done for all patients. If LFTs are abnormal, hepatitis serologies should also be done.

Further diagnostic testing may be suggested by the initial history, exam, and labs.

If not, a CT scan of the abdomen should be the next diagnostic step to pick up two of the most common causes of FUO: intraabdominal abscess and lymphoma. ⓑ

Lower-extremity venous duplex is recommended if previously mentioned studies are negative because DVT has caused 2–6% of FUO in recent series. ⓑ

A temporal artery biopsy should be considered early in the evaluation of older patients because giant cell arteritis is a common cause of FUO in this population. ⓑ

Endocarditis causes 1–5% of FUO. Although echocardiography has not been studied specifically in the setting of FUO, the sensitivity of a transthoracic echocardiogram for endocarditis is ∼65%, whereas that of transesophageal echocardiography approaches 100%.

Nuclear imaging studies, such as tagged white cell or gallium scans, are insensitive but may reveal an unsuspected locus of infection. ⓑ

Liver biopsy may yield a diagnosis even in the setting of normal LFTs and radiographic imaging; if no other diagnostic possibilities are raised by the previously mentioned studies, a liver biopsy may be the next step, particularly if the patient is deteriorating. ⓑ

Discharge Planning:

The patient may be discharged prior to arriving at a diagnosis if clinically stable and close outpatient follow-up is arranged.

If a diagnosis has not been made, the temperature should be measured and recorded several times per day, and the patient should be instructed to call or come in for any new symptoms.

Special Considerations:

Consultation with infectious disease, hematology/oncology, or rheumatology should be guided by initial lab studies and clinical impression of the most likely cause of FUO.

Reference

Mourad O, Palda V, Detsky AS: A comprehensive evidence based approach to fever of unknown origin. *Arch Intern Med* 163:545–551, 2003.

Seizure

Seizures are caused by abnormal, synchronized excitation of cortical neurons. Seizures can be partial onset (focal excitation) or generalized onset (diffuse excitation), and either simple (not affecting consciousness) or complex (affecting consciousness to any degree). Complex seizures are often followed by a postictal state with somnolence and confusion lasting from several minutes to several hours.

Epilepsy describes recurrent seizures in which the cause is not easily reversed. Provoked seizures have reversible causes, most commonly:

- Hypoglycemia
- Fever
- Medications
- Alcohol withdrawal
- Acute trauma
- Central nervous system (CNS) infection

Provoked seizures generally do not require long-term treatment, except of the underlying cause.

Patients with first-time seizures who are neurologically normal and can be monitored closely at home may not require inpatient admission if they are reliable to follow-up. Other patients with first-time seizures are typically admitted to the hospital.

Recurrent epileptic seizures similar in quality and frequency to the patient's previous seizures do not usually require

---

❹Recommendation based on consistent and good quality patient-oriented evidence. ❺ Recommendation based on inconsistent or limited quality patient-oriented evidence. ❻ Recommendation based on usual practice, consensus, opinion, disease-oriented evidence, or case series for studies of diagnosis, treatment, and prevention of screening.

extensive work-up or inpatient admission. The most common reasons for recurrent seizures in patients with epilepsy are:

- Medically refractory disease, which affects up to 40% of patients in some references
- Subtherapeutic medication levels from noncompliance

Status epilepticus is a life-threatening emergency (mortality 5–22%) and always requires admission, usually to ICU-level care.

These orders are for a 25-year-old man with poor social support and first-time seizure.

Admit to: Floor

Most patients admitted with seizure are stable enough for a neurology or medical floor. Those with status epilepticus are typically admitted to the ICU.

Diagnosis: Seizure

Condition: Stable

Although most patients with seizure are stable, those with status epilepticus have 5–20% mortality and should be listed in "critical" condition.

Vital Signs:

Routine, with O$_2$ saturation

Patients receiving IV antiepileptic medications, which can cause arrhythmia, should be monitored on telemetry during infusion. Hypoxia and hyperthermia should be aggressively treated because these may provoke seizure.

Activity: Fall and Seizure Precautions

Patients at high risk for recurrent seizures should get up with assistance. Bed rails are often padded to reduce the risk of injury. Other protective equipment, such as bedside foam landing strips, should be used if available.

N ursing:

Neurologic checks q 1 hour for 2 hours, q 2 hours for 4 hours, and then q 4 hours
Check capillary blood glucose (CBG) q 4 hours

Initially, frequent checks are done to ensure the neurologic status is not deteriorating.

Hypoglycemia can provoke seizures, and blood glucose should be checked frequently in patients with treated diabetes.

Video electroencephalogram (EEG) may be useful to confirm or disprove a seizure etiology for altered mental status or shaking.

D iet: Routine

IV Fluids: Heplock IV

Hypotonic solutions can lead to cerebral edema, so they should be used with care.

M edications:

Diazepam 5 mg IV now. Repeat in 5 minutes for ongoing seizure

The treatment of choice for an ongoing seizure is a benzodiazepine. Options include:

- Diazepam 5–10 mg bolus at 5-minute intervals
- Lorazepam 2–5 mg bolus at 5-minute intervals
- Midazolam at 0.2 mg/kg bolus followed by 0.75–10 µg/kg/min

Phenobarbital at 15–20 mg/kg, given at a maximal rate of 100 mg/min, is also effective for treatment of ongoing seizures but carries a higher risk of hypoventilation, hypotension, and prolonged sedation.

Phenytoin IV (15–20 mg/kg at 50 mg/min, with cardiac monitoring for arrhythmias) and fosphenytoin IV (15–20 mg/kg at 150 mg/min) loading usually achieve serum phenytoin levels > 10 mg/L within minutes of infusion. IM loading of fosphenytoin (same as IV dose) achieves levels > 10 mg/L within 1 hour. Oral loading of phenytoin (15–20 mg/kg divided over three doses, each dose separated by 2 hours) results in a therapeutic level 3–8 hours after initial ingestion. Valproate can be loaded IV (15 mg/kg over 60 minutes) or orally (20 mg/kg loading dose). Frequently a total of 30–40 mg/kg may be required to achieve therapeutic levels in the first few hours.

Propofol may be used in refractory status epilepticus. If paralytics are required for airway protection or ventilation, aggressive treatment of clinically inapparent but ongoing seizures is required, along with continuous EEG monitoring.

Phenytoin, valproate, phenobarbital, and carbamazepine can be used for seizure prophylaxis. Newer antiepileptic drugs are generally more expensive and less studied but have fewer side effects and a wider therapeutic window (and therefore have less need for drug monitoring). Examples include gabapentin, lamotrigine, topiramate, tiagabine, levetiracetam, oxcarbazepine, and zonisamide.

The decision to start long-term antiepileptic drug therapy for first-time seizures should be made individually for each patient. Immediate therapy for first-time seizures was recently shown to reduce seizure occurrence over the near term but did not affect long-term remission (76% of patients were seizure free between years 3–5, regardless of whether they received initial therapy). **B**

Labs and Diagnostic Studies:

Chem 7, calcium, magnesium
Blood alcohol level, urine toxicology, and antiepileptic
   medication levels, thyroid-stimulating hormone (TSH),
   beta-human chorionic gonadotropin (HCG)
Noncontrast head CT
Anticipate lumbar puncture after CT
EEG in AM

Seizures may be provoked by hypoglycemia, hyponatremia, hypomagnesemia, hypercalcemia, or uremia. Tonic-clonic seizures can result in a transient lactic acidosis due to muscle contraction, so do not be surprised by a low serum bicarbonate. ❸

Antiepileptic drugs, including phenytoin, carbamazepine, valproic acid, and phenobarbital, have reference levels that can be followed.

Hyperthyroidism has rarely been reported to cause seizures.

Many antiepileptic drugs are teratogenic, and a pregnancy test should be done in females prior to administration.

Noncontrast head CT assesses for intracranial mass lesion, evidence of cerebrovascular disease, trauma, or spontaneous intracranial hemorrhage as a cause of seizure.

Lumbar puncture should be performed only after a space-occupying mass is excluded on CT and can help diagnose CNS infection, subarachnoid hemorrhage, or meningeal neoplasm as a cause of seizure. Lumbar puncture is especially important for patients who are immunocompromised or have signs of infection or meningeal irritation.

Cerebrospinal fluid (CSF) should be sent for cell count and differential, protein, glucose, and xanthochromia. Consider bacterial, viral, fungal, and mycobacterial cultures; viral polymerase chain reactions (PCRs) (e.g., herpes simplex virus [HSV], varicella-zoster virus [VZV]), and/or cryptococcal antigen (Ag) depending on patient presentation.

ECG may identify arrhythmia or ischemia as a cause of cerebral hypoxia.

EEG is often helpful but is not always needed and is imperfectly sensitive and specific.

MRI is generally more sensitive than CT in identifying masses, blood, congenital anomalies, vascular lesions, or infarct. MRI can be considered if other work-up is inconclusive for a cause of seizure. ❸

D ischarge Planning:

Seizures not provoked by a correctable systemic process should be evaluated by a neurologist, in most cases prior to discharge. ❸

Driving restrictions vary by state but should be discussed with all patients. Some states have mandatory physician reporting to the Department of Motor Vehicles (DMV).

Unsupervised baths/swimming, exposure to heights (climbing ladders, roof repair), and operation of heavy machinery should be discouraged until discussed with a neurologist and the likelihood of seizure recurrence is assessed.

If new drugs are started, drug levels and toxicities should be monitored closely after follow-up. Patients should receive detailed information about the drug interactions (e.g., with warfarin and oral contraceptives) and side effects that are common with antiepileptic medications.

Encourage and provide affected patients with resources for substance abuse management.

S pecial Considerations:

Patients with seizure may suffer occult trauma that is not obvious at presentation because of altered mental status. A careful exam and imaging of painful body parts can help avoid missing occult injury.

References

Clinical policy: Critical issues in the evaluation and management of adult patients presenting to the emergency department with seizures. *Ann Emerg Med* 43:605–625, 2004.

Marson A, Jacoby A, Johnson A, et al: Immediate versus deferred antiepileptic drug treatment for early epilepsy and single seizures: A randomized controlled trial. *Lancet* 365:2007–2013, 2005.

Acute Ischemic Stroke

Stroke, defined as neurologic dysfunction of sudden onset and probable vascular cause, is a leading cause of death in the United States. The majority of strokes are ischemic, caused by embolic or thrombotic occlusion of a cerebral vessel; intracranial hemorrhage is much less common. Emergent brain imaging, usually with noncontrast head CT, differentiates ischemic from hemorrhagic stroke.

These orders are for an 80-year-old man with longstanding severe hypertension who awoke this morning with difficulty speaking and weakness of the right arm.

A dmit to: Floor

Almost all patients with acute stroke should be admitted to the hospital, both to facilitate timely evaluation and to assess functional status and plan for future care. The severity of neurologic symptoms dictates initial triage to the ICU or to the ward, preferably a ward with expertise in stroke care. Patients with airway compromise, depressed level of consciousness, severe hypertension, and possible arrhythmia or myocardial ischemia should be admitted to the ICU or a step-down unit with telemetry and close monitoring capabilities. More stable patients may be admitted to the floor. ◉

D iagnosis: Acute Ischemic Stroke

C ondition: Guarded

Despite recent advances in stroke therapy and improvement in outcomes, cerebrovascular disease is still the third leading cause of death, and patients presenting with acute stroke are at risk for medical and neurologic complications of the stroke as well as early recurrent stroke. Patients requiring ICU admission are critical. ◉

V ital Signs:

Every 4 hours. Neurologic checks q 2 hours for the first 24 hours, then q 4 hours. Call for temperature > 38°C, SBP > 200 mmHg or < 120 mmHg, HR > 100 bpm

Monitor neurologic status closely over the first few days following stroke. Neurologic symptoms may improve, but patients may also suffer recurrent stroke or hemorrhagic transformation (especially with thrombolytic or anticoagulant therapy). ◉

Hypertension, often severe, is common in acute stroke, although its optimal management is not clear. There is no evidence that lowering blood pressure is beneficial, and lower blood pressure could decrease perfusion of ischemia but still viable areas of brain. Therefore, most authorities recommend that in the absence of end-organ manifestations of severe hypertension (i.e., pulmonary edema, myocardial ischemia, acute renal failure) no antihypertensives be given unless SBP > 220 mmHg, or diastolic blood pressure (DBP) > 120 mmHg. Severe hypertension will usually improve without therapy. **©**

Fever is deleterious in acute stroke and should be aggressively treated. **Ⓑ**

A llergies: NKDA

A ctivity: Bedrest Until Initial Physical Therapy Assessment Done, then Mobilize ASAP as Guided by Physical Therapy. Strict Fall Precautions

Mobilize patients as early as is safe to do so, with the assistance of trained personnel. Early mobilization may maintain function and help avoid deep vein thrombosis (DVT) and decubitus ulcers. Prolonged, unnecessary bedrest should be avoided. **©**

N ursing:

Supplemental oxygen to maintain O_2 saturation > 93%
Check capillary blood glucose q 6 hours

Patients with hypoxia should receive supplemental oxygen, but there is no evidence that oxygen is helpful in patients with normal oxygenation.

Hyperglycemia in acute ischemic stroke has been associated with worse outcomes, although this is at least partly due to the greater likelihood of hyperglycemia in patients with more severe strokes. A study of more intensive control of hyperglycemia in stroke is being done, but for now, it should be managed as in any acute medical illness (*see* Diabetes Management, pp 275–280). **©**

Diet: NPO Until Swallow Evaluation Performed. Then Begin Heart Healthy Diet as Recommended by Speech Pathology

Any patient with altered level of consciousness, cranial nerve dysfunction, inability to cough on command, or complaint of dysphagia should be kept NPO until swallow function is evaluated, ideally by a speech pathologist, to prevent aspiration and pneumonia. If the patient is alert and has intact cranial nerve function, including the ability to cough on command and a normal gag reflex, the ability to swallow can be screened with a small amount of water. If this causes any coughing or a "wet" voice, the patient should be made NPO until more formal swallow evaluation. ◉

A speech pathologist can also make recommendations for safe food texture and eating practices to minimize any risk of aspiration.

If the patient will be NPO for longer than 1 or 2 days, consider placing a nasogastric feeding tube, both to provide enteral nutrition and to provide a route to administer oral medications. Because swallowing function may improve in the days following stroke, a percutaneous gastrostomy (PEG) tube is usually not considered until after an initial period of recovery. ◉

IV Fluids: Normal Saline (NS) at 50 mL/h. Avoid Glucose-Containing Solutions Whenever Possible. Heplock IV When Taking Adequate PO

Hyperglycemia has been associated with, although it does not clearly cause, adverse outcomes in patients with stroke, so dextrose-containing IV fluids should generally be avoided unless a continuous insulin infusion is prescribed. ◉

Excessive IV fluids or hyponatremia could theoretically worsen cerebral edema in the area of the stroke. If the patient is not able to swallow, order IV fluid sufficient to avoid volume depletion but not so much as to cause volume overload. Some physicians prefer isotonic fluid because there is less risk of developing hyponatremia than with $\frac{1}{2}$ NS. ◉

Medications:

Aspirin 325 mg PO qd
Acetaminophen 650 mg q 6 hours for 48 hours to prevent fever
Docusate 100 mg PO bid
Heparin 5000 units SQ q 8 hours

The most urgent medication to consider in acute stroke is tissue plasminogen activator (tPA), which can improve neurologic outcomes, although not mortality, in a carefully selected minority of patients with stroke. Most patients with stroke either present too late or have contraindications to the use of tPA. tPA is indicated only for patients with a clinical diagnosis of stroke, with onset of symptoms within 3 hours of tPA administration, after a CT scan has been performed with no evidence of hemorrhage or edema. Contraindications to the use of tPA include sustained severe hypertension, thrombocytopenia or abnormal clotting, hyperglycemia or hypoglycemia, minor or rapidly improving symptoms, prior hemorrhagic stroke, stroke or head injury in the past 3 months, major surgery in the past 2 weeks, gastrointestinal (GI) bleeding in the past 3 weeks, recent myocardial infarction (MI), and coma. ◉

Because of the significant risk of bleeding and hemorrhagic transformation of stroke, tPA is typically administered in specialized stroke centers in consultation with a neurologist experienced in stroke care. As more hospitals develop stroke centers and public awareness of the emergent nature

of neurologic symptoms grows, the number of patients treated with tPA is likely to grow.

If tPA is given, the patient's vital signs and neurologic
status must be monitored very closely in an ICU or stroke
unit. Hypertension must be controlled, maintaining SBP
< 180 mmHg and DBP < 105 mmHg, to reduce the chance
of hemorrhagic transformation. Note that goals for blood
pressure control are very different for tPA-treated and untreated patients. Any change in neurologic status should be
reported immediately.

Antiplatelet therapy should be prescribed for all patients,
although it should not be started for at least 24 hours following administration for those treated with tPA. Aspirin
reduces the risk of recurrent stroke, and possibly death, in
treated patients. **Ⓐ**

Other antiplatelet drugs, including clopidogrel (Plavix)
and dipyridamole combined with aspirin (Aggrenox) are mar-
ginally more effective than aspirin, but substantially more
expensive. If a patient was not on aspirin prior to the stroke,
aspirin should be prescribed. If the patient was on aspirin,
alternate antiplatelet therapy could be considered. **Ⓒ**

Fever in patients with acute ischemic stroke has been
associated with worse neurologic outcomes and increased
mortality. Acetaminophen can be prescribed to prevent
fever. If it cannot be given by mouth, it may be given via a
nasogastric tube or as a rectal suppository. **Ⓑ**

Venous thromboembolism is common in patients with
acute stroke, and pulmonary embolism accounts for 10%
of deaths following stroke. DVT prophylaxis should be
prescribed for all patients. SQ heparin can be prescribed
immediately for patients who have not been treated with
tPA but should not be started until 24 hours after administration for those who have. Sequential compression devices
can be substituted for patients with contraindications to
heparin. **Ⓐ**

There is no clear benefit to early, urgent anticoagulation for most patients with acute ischemic stroke, including those with presumed cardioembolic stroke, and IV heparin increases the risk of hemorrhagic transformation, especially in patients with large strokes. **Ⓐ**

Consideration could be given to heparin anticoagulation for patients with presumed basilar artery thrombosis or cardioembolic stroke, in consultation with a neurologist. **Ⓒ**

Warfarin anticoagulation is indicated to prevent recurrent stroke in patients with atrial fibrillation, but the timing of initiation of warfarin will depend on the severity of the stroke. **Ⓐ**

Constipation is common in stroke patients, and a bowel program should be prescribed.

Although control of hypertension is not a part of treatment of most acute stroke, it is important in the long term. Gradual control of hypertension over a period of weeks is the usual recommendation. The addition of a less potent antihypertensive, such as hydrochlorothiazide, should be considered as the patient approaches discharge. **Ⓒ**

In follow-up, an angiotensin-converting enzyme (ACE) inhibitor should be added to improve long-term vascular outcomes. **Ⓐ**

As discharge approaches, lipid therapy should be initiated (typically with a statin), with a goal low-density lipoprotein (LDL) of < 100 mg/dL. **Ⓐ**

Labs and Diagnostic Studies:

Noncontrast CT of the head, complete blood count (CBC) with platelet count, prothrombin time (PT), partial thromboplastin time (PTT), Chem 7, liver function tests (LFTs), ECG

Carotid duplex, echocardiogram in AM

Daily CBC with platelets, Chem 7

After rapid initial evaluation and stabilization, brain imaging is indicated for all patients presenting with acute stroke, especially those who are candidates for tPA. The goal for tPA candidates is imaging and interpretation within 45 minutes of arrival at the emergency room. **Ⓐ**

Noncontrast CT identifies all patients with hemorrhagic stroke who cannot be treated with tPA, and it can identify some nonstroke causes of neurologic symptoms. However, CT scan is relatively insensitive for small or early strokes. **Ⓑ**

Contrast is used if tumor or infection is a significant consideration. MRI with diffusion-weighted imaging is more sensitive and is being used at some centers for imaging of suspected acute stroke. **Ⓑ**

CBC with platelets and assessment of coagulation is done to assess risk for hemorrhage and prior to therapy with tPA. Chem 7 and LFTs should also be done in all patients presenting with stroke. **Ⓒ**

Cardiovascular assessment is an important part of the evaluation of patients with ischemic stroke because the heart and blood vessels are a source of emboli and the risk of concurrent cardiac disease is high. In addition to physical examination, ECG should be performed in all patients. If ECG shows evidence of acute ischemia, cardiac monitoring, serial cardiac enzymes, and consultation with a cardiologist are warranted. **Ⓒ**

Because timely treatment of symptomatic carotid stenosis can reduce the risk of recurrent stroke, all patients should have imaging of the carotid arteries, usually with carotid duplex ultrasonography first. **Ⓐ**

Echocardiography should be performed in patients with presumed embolic stroke to look for cardiac source of emboli and left ventricular dysfunction. The choice of transthoracic versus transesophageal echo is controversial. Transesophageal echo reveals more abnormalities but has not been shown to change outcomes, so transthoracic echo is a reasonable choice for most patients. Consider trans-esophageal echo for younger patients and those with no identified cause for stroke. **B**

Discharge Planning:

Patients must be neurologically stable, able to eat or have a feeding tube in place, and have a safe discharge destination arranged prior to discharge.

Physical therapy and occupational therapy consults should be obtained on the first hospital day. Therapists can assess functional status and postdischarge therapy and equipment needs and make recommendations for post-discharge destination—acute care rehabilitation versus skilled nursing facility for subacute rehabilitation versus home. **C**

Social work should also be consulted for assistance with discharge planning immediately because many patients will need placement or home health services. **C**

Speech pathologist consultation will guide the choice of diet versus enteral feeding.

At discharge, a statin should be started if the LDL is > 100 mg/dL. **A**

Patients who smoke should be educated on cessation and offered antismoking aids. **A**

Follow-up should be arranged within 2 weeks.

Special Considerations:

Neurology consultation should be considered for all patients with stroke and is particularly important when a patient is eligible for treatment with tPA.

A decline in neurologic status should prompt a repeat head CT, seeking hemorrhagic transformation (especially in a patient treated with tPA) or edema.

References

Adams HP, Adams RJ, Brott T, et al: Guidelines for the early management of patients with ischemic stroke: A scientific statement from the Stroke Council of the American Stroke Association. *Stroke* 34:1056–1083, 2003.

Albers GW, Amarenco P, Easton JD, et al: Antithrombotic therapy for acute ischemic stroke. The Seventh ACCP Conference on Antithrombotic and Thrombolytic Therapy. *Chest* 126:483S–512S, 2004.

Alcohol Withdrawal

Alcohol withdrawal is defined as two or more of:

- Autonomic hyperactivity
- Tremor
- Insomnia
- Hallucinations
- Nausea or vomiting
- Psychomotor agitation
- Anxiety
- Grand mal seizure

developing within several hours to several days of the abrupt cessation of heavy, prolonged alcohol use.

Patients presenting to the emergency room with symptoms of mild alcohol withdrawal are sometimes treated as outpatients or referred to a detox facility if available; inpatient admission may be required for patients with more severe symptoms and for those with comorbid medical or surgical illness, who are at higher risk of severe withdrawal.

Many patients admitted for unrelated medical and surgical problems suffer alcohol dependence and are also at risk for withdrawal when they stop drinking abruptly.

Alcohol withdrawal may present within 24 hours of the last drink, but symptoms typically peak 48–72 hours after admission.

These orders are for a 61-year-old man with a long history of alcohol use, presenting with 1 day of nausea, vomiting, and fever.

A dmit to: Floor

Most patients with alcohol withdrawal can be managed on a medical floor. Patients with severe alcohol withdrawal, characterized by marked autonomic hyperactivity and hallucinations, may require ICU care for cardiac monitoring, frequent (or continuous) IV benzodiazepines, and, rarely, intubation and paralysis.

D iagnosis: Alcohol Withdrawal

C ondition: Stable

If recognized and treated appropriately, most patients with alcohol withdrawal recover over several days to 1 week.

V ital Signs:

Check vital signs q 2 hours × 4, then q 4 hours
Call MD for temperature > 38.5 °C, HR > 110 bpm,
   SBP > 180 mmHg

Autonomic hyperactivity can cause tachycardia, hypertension, and fever.

A llergies: NKDA

Activity: Bedrest, Fall Precautions. Ambulate with Assistance Only If Able to Safely Stand

Patients with alcohol withdrawal are often agitated and impulsive and are at risk for falls and injury.

Nursing:

Perform Clinical Institute Withdrawal Assessment for Alcohol (CIWAA) revised scale on admission, q 2 hours × 4, then if score < 9, q 4 hours

The CIWAA scale is a reliable, validated tool for assessing the severity of alcohol withdrawal and can help guide treatment with benzodiazepines. Patients are assessed regularly for:

- Nausea and vomiting
- Tremor
- Paroxysmal sweats
- Anxiety
- Agitation
- Tactile disturbances
- Auditory disturbances
- Visual disturbances
- Headache
- Orientation and clouding of sensorium

Points are assigned on a 0–7 scale for each item.

Diet: Diet as Tolerated. Please Assist with Meals

If the patient is sedated or has a decreased level of consciousness, oral intake should be withheld to avoid aspiration.

IV Fluids: NS 250 mL/h for 1 Liter, Followed by D5 $\frac{1}{2}$ NS at 100 mL/h

Volume depletion should be corrected and maintenance fluids administered until the patient is able to eat and drink.

Medications

**Chlordiazepoxide 25 mg PO q 2–4 hours prn CIWAA
score 9–15**
Chlordiazepoxide 50 mg PO q 2–4 hours prn CIWAA score > 15
Thiamine 100 mg PO qd for 3 days
Multivitamin PO qd
Folic acid 1 mg PO qd

Benzodiazepines are the treatment of choice for alcohol withdrawal. **Ⓐ**

Chlordiazepoxide (Librium) is a long-acting oral benzodiazepine that is effective for most patients.

Lorazepam has a shorter half-life and is often preferred for elderly patients and those with significant liver disease, who may metabolize drugs more slowly. Lorazepam may also be given IV or IM for patients unable to take oral medications. **Ⓑ**

A symptom-triggered benzodiazepine dosing regimen based on the CIWAA score has been shown to be safe and effective and to decrease the duration of treatment and the amount of drug administered compared with older, fixed-dose regimens. **Ⓐ**

The CIWAA score is assessed by the nursing staff at admission and repeated in 2 hours if it is 9 or more and in 4 hours if it is 8 or less.

Patients with alcohol abuse often suffer nutritional deficiency. Administration of glucose (in IV fluids) may precipitate Wernicke's encephalopathy in patients with unrecognized thiamine deficiency; therefore, thiamine supplementation is appropriate for patients admitted with alcohol withdrawal. **Ⓑ**

Magnesium deficiency is also common in alcoholism and should be corrected as low levels can lower the seizure threshold. **Ⓒ**

Labs and Diagnostic Studies:

Admit: CBC, Chem 7, calcium, magnesium, phosphate, liver function tests, international normalized ratio (INR), urinalysis (UA), blood cultures × 2, chest x-ray (CXR), ECG
Daily Chem 7, magnesium

Admit labs should assess for:

- Any illness precipitating alcohol withdrawal, especially infection
- Other effects of alcohol abuse; for example, cirrhosis, hepatitis, or electrolyte or nutritional deficiency
- Complications of alcohol withdrawal, such as cardiac ischemia due to tachycardia

Other labs may be indicated based on initial history, exam, and labs.

Discharge Planning:

Patients with alcohol withdrawal are typically discharged when:

- Their sensorium has cleared.
- They are no longer requiring prn doses of benzodiazepines.
- They are able to take oral food and fluids.
- Other medical illnesses have resolved or stabilized.

All patients admitted with alcohol withdrawal should meet with a social worker or substance abuse counselor to discuss their addiction and review available resources, such as Alcoholic Anonymous and outpatient or inpatient addiction treatment.

The physician should also emphasize the importance of alcohol cessation in discharge education.

Special Considerations:

All patients admitted to the hospital should be screened for alcohol dependence before developing symptoms of withdrawal. Patients with self-reported heavy alcohol use can be regularly monitored with the CIWAA scale, and treatment initiated promptly if significant withdrawal symptoms develop.

Depression commonly coexists with alcohol abuse, and one may hamper the patient's ability to cope with the other. Psychiatric consultation may be helpful for patients with both diagnoses.

References

Daeppen JB, Gache P, Landry U, et al: Symptom triggered versus fixed schedule benzodiazepine dosing for alcohol withdrawal. A randomized controlled trial. *Arch Intern Med* 162:1117–1121, 2002.

Kosten TR, O'Connor PG: Management of drug and alcohol withdrawal. *N Engl J Med* 348:1786–1795, 2003.

Ntais C, Pakos E, Kyzas P, Ioannidis JP: Benzodiazepines for alcohol withdrawal. *Cochrane Database Syst Rev* 3: 2005CD005063.

8

Acute Renal Failure

The most common causes of acute renal failure (ARF) are:

- Acute tubular necrosis, most often due to sepsis or hypotension
- Prerenal azotemia due to volume depletion *or* ineffective circulating volume, as in heart failure or cirrhosis
- Nephrotoxic drugs
- Urinary tract obstruction

Less common causes include glomerulonephritis, vasculitis, and atheroembolic disease.

The initial orders focus on establishing the cause, correcting volume depletion if present, and monitoring for and treating complications of ARF.

These orders are for a 68-year-old woman with mild chronic renal insufficiency and a recent bout of gastroenteritis, admitted with creatinine of 4.8 mg/dL.

Admit to: Telemetry Floor

Patients with ARF and hyperkalemia should be monitored on telemetry.

Diagnosis: Acute Renal Failure

Condition: Guarded

Most patients admitted with renal failure have comorbid illnesses, often severe. The mortality rate of ICU patients who require dialysis for ARF is > 60%.

Ⓐ Recommendation based on consistent and good quality patient-oriented evidence. **Ⓑ** Recommendation based on inconsistent or limited quality patient-oriented evidence. **Ⓒ** Recommendation based on usual practice, consensus, opinion, disease-oriented evidence, or case series for studies of diagnosis, treatment, and prevention of screening.

V ital Signs:

Routine
Check orthostatic vital signs on admission and once per shift

Hypotension is common in patients with renal failure and volume overload. Positive orthostatic vital signs support volume depletion as the cause of prerenal ARF, as does low jugular venous pressure.

A llergies: Routine

A ctivity: Ad Lib

N ursing:

Place Foley catheter
Strict inputs and outputs (I/Os)
Daily weights
Call for urinary output (UO) < 200 mL/shift, O_2 saturation < 92%

In patients with acute tubular necrosis, oliguria (< 500 mL urine/24 hours) is associated with worse prognosis for renal recovery.

Anuria (< 50 mL urine/day) is rare and should suggest shock, complete urinary obstruction, and bilateral renal artery obstruction as possible causes of ARF.

A Foley catheter can both:

- Assist in collection of urine for laboratory studies
- Exclude bladder outlet obstruction (e.g., due to prostatic hypertrophy) as the cause of ARF.

However, the catheter should be removed as soon as possible to decrease the risk of urinary tract infection (UTI).

Volume status should be followed very carefully in ARF: Inadequate volume resuscitation will delay recovery from prerenal azotemia, but excessive volume in an oliguric patient may worsen pulmonary and peripheral edema and hasten the need for dialysis. **Ⓒ**

D iet: Renal Diet

At most hospitals, a renal diet has low sodium, low potassium, and low phosphate. Patients without hyperkalemia or hyperphosphatemia and with good UO may be kept on a regular diet.

IV Fluids: Normal Saline (NS) 250 mL/h for 3 Hours, then Call MD to Reassess

IV fluid orders will be guided by the initial differential diagnosis and volume status. If the patient is felt to be volume depleted, isotonic fluid should be administered until euvolemic. If the patient is not felt to be volume depleted, IV should be heplocked.

Frequent reassessment of volume status is the key to avoiding iatrogenic volume overload in patients with presumed prerenal azotemia. Order 1–1.5 L of isotonic fluid, then reassess volume status by checking HR, BP, orthostatic vital signs, UO, and jugular venous pressure. Continue to administer isotonic fluid until the patient is euvolemic. **Ⓒ**

M edications:

Calcium carbonate 1000 mg PO tid with meals

Calcium carbonate, calcium carbonate, or another oral phosphate binder should be initiated in patients who are eating and have elevated serum phosphate. These drugs bind to phosphate in the gut and prevent absorption. They are not useful in patients who have no oral intake. **Ⓑ**

Review the patient's outpatient medications very carefully, and stop all that are nephrotoxic, especially nonsteroidal anti-inflammatory drugs (NSAIDs), angiotensin-converting enzyme (ACE) inhibitors and angiotensin receptor blockers. ❽

Correct the dose of all other renally cleared medications for the patient's renal failure, using the calculated glomerular filtration rate (GFR).

Labs and Diagnostic Studies

Urinalysis (UA) and microscopic evaluation, urine sodium and creatinine, Chem 7, complete blood count (CBC), calcium, magnesium, and phosphate, renal ultrasound

A careful evaluation of the urine sediment is critical in evaluating ARF. Muddy brown casts suggest acute tubular necrosis, red cell casts or dysmorphic red cells suggest glomerulonephritis, and urine eosinophils or large numbers of white cells suggest interstitial nephritis. The sediment is usually bland in prerenal azotemia.

The urine sodium and creatinine can be used to calculate the fractional excretion of sodium (FeNa) with the following equation:

FeNa% = (Urine sodium × plasma creatinine) / (Plasma sodium × urine creatinine) × 100

A FeNa less than 1% supports a diagnosis of prerenal azotemia.

If the cause of ARF is not clear after this initial evaluation, a renal ultrasound should be performed to assess for obstruction and other renal abnormalities. ❽

If the diagnosis remains unclear, any of an extensive battery of serologic tests may be performed, but these should generally not be ordered for all patients admitted with ARF.

Discharge Planning:

Discharge planning will depend on the diagnosis. Patients with volume depletion and prerenal azotemia are typically improved and ready for discharge within 2 or 3 days, whereas those with acute tubular necrosis often require dialysis for 1–3 weeks prior to recovery of renal function. If persistent renal insufficiency is present at discharge, the patient should be instructed to follow a renal diet and weigh himself or herself daily at home and to call the physician if he or she gains more than 3–4 pounds (a sign of volume overload).

Special Considerations:

Indications for acute hemodialysis:

- Acidemia
- Electrolyte abnormalities, especially hyperkalemia
- Ingestion
- Overload (volume)

Uremia symptoms, including lethargy, mental status changes, seizures, asterixis, uremic pericarditis, vomiting

Reference

Dursun B, Edelstein BL: Acute renal failure. *Am J Kidney Dis* 45:614–618, 2005.

Hyperkalemia

The most common causes of hyperkalemia are chronic renal failure, often with missed dialysis, and medications, including ACE inhibitors, angiotensin receptor blockers, spironolactone, triamterene, NSAIDs and high-dose tri-methoprim-sulfamethoxazole. Commercial salt substitutes also contain substantial amounts of potassium.

These orders are for a 42-year-old man with heart failure and renal insufficiency, recently started on spironolactone in addition to his ACE inhibitor.

A dmit to: Telemetry Floor

Patients with significant hyperkalemia are at risk for life-threatening arrhythmia and must be admitted for close follow-up and cardiac monitoring. If the potassium remains elevated or ECG changes persist despite initial therapy in the emergency room, ICU admission is warranted.

D iagnosis: Hyperkalemia

C ondition: Guarded

Significant hyperkalemia (> 6 Eq/L) can cause life-threatening arrhythmias.

V ital Signs: Routine

Hyperkalemia does not result in hemodynamic instability unless an associated arrhythmia develops.

A llergies: NKDA

A ctivity: As Tolerated

Patients with ECG changes should be on bedrest because of the risk of falls with arrhythmia.

N ursing:

ECG on admission and with changes in potassium level
Strict I/Os

An ECG should be done immediately on recognition of hyperkalemia. Peaked T waves are the earliest sign of hyperkalemia, followed by prolonged PR and QRS intervals, which may progress to sine wave and ventricular fibrillation or asystole. Although a normal ECG is reassuring, it does not obviate the need to increase potassium excretion from the body. ☉

It is important to chart a patient's intake and UO because decreased UO can perpetuate hyperkalemia or point to a possible cause. ☉

Ⓓiet: Renal (Low Potassium)

Potassium is found in many foods, particularly in citrus fruits, melons, tomatoes, and salt substitutes. Lower concentrations are found in many foods. Nutrition consultation for diet education may be helpful in preventing further episodes of hyperkalemia. ☉

ⒾⱽFluids: NS 200 mL/h for 6 Hours

In a patient who is not anuric, NS increases urinary flow, which increases potassium excretion. Do not use IV fluids to treat hyperkalemia in dialysis patients, who will simply become volume overloaded. ☉

Ⓜedications:

Calcium gluconate 10 mL of 10% solution IV over 2 minutes
Regular insulin 10 units IV, administered with 1 amp of D50
Nebulized albuterol × 1 now
Sodium polystyrene sulfate (Kayexalate) 15 g PO qid—first dose ASAP
Furosemide (Lasix) 40 mg IV × 1 now

Calcium gluconate stabilizes cardiac cell membranes to prevent arrhythmia. It should be given regardless of serum calcium levels. ECG changes should improve within 3 minutes; if not, the dose can be repeated after 5 minutes. The effect of calcium gluconate lasts 30–60 minutes. Ⓑ

Insulin shifts potassium into cells, decreasing serum potassium. It should be administered with 1 amp of D50 if serum glucose is < 250 mg/dL. An effect can be seen after 20 minutes and should last 4–6 hours. The effect of insulin is prolonged in patients with end-stage renal disease (ESRD), so capillary blood glucose should be followed closely. **Ⓑ**

Nebulized albuterol also shifts potassium into cells, but its effect is antagonized by beta blockers and it is ineffective in many patients. It may be used as an adjunct in severe hyperkalemia but is not recommended as the only treatment of hyperkalemia. **Ⓑ**

Sodium bicarbonate IV can also be used to shift potassium intracellularly, but it is ineffective in some patients, causes volume overload and hypertension, and is falling out of favor. It may be used for urgent treatment of hyperkalemia in addition to other measures, especially for patients with acidosis. **Ⓑ**

All of the previously discussed therapies work quickly but are temporary; potassium must also be eliminated from the body via the gastrointestinal (GI) tract, kidneys, or dialysis. Sodium polystyrene sulfate (Kayexalate) is a resin that binds potassium in the GI tract. The resin is mixed with sorbitol, which causes diarrhea and additional stool potassium loss. It is modestly effective in decreasing serum potassium. It can also be given as an enema and may work faster.

Furosemide will accelerate renal sodium losses *if* the patient is not anuric. Patients with severe hyperkalemia and renal failure may require emergent hemodialysis. **Ⓒ**

Remember that medications commonly contribute to hyperkalemia. Hold all potassium supplements, ACE inhibitors, angiotensin receptor blockers, and potassium-sparing diuretics. Consider other medications as possible causes, including NSAIDs, beta blockers, and trimethoprim. **Ⓒ**

Labs and Diagnostic Studies:

Admission: stat repeat potassium, CBC, UA, urinary potassium

Repeat potassium in 4 hours

A finding of hyperkalemia may be spurious, usually due to hemolysis during the process of blood collection. If a patient has no clinical or ECG findings of hyperkalemia, the measurement should be repeated with a new specimen prior to initiating therapy. **ⓒ**

Discharge Planning

Patients with ESRD should be aware of the location and time of next scheduled dialysis run.

Nutrition should be consulted prior to discharge for education about low-potassium diet.

Potassium levels and renal function should be stable prior to discharge.

The discharge medications should be reviewed carefully for any that could contribute to hyperkalemia. Alternate medications should be considered whenever possible.

Special Considerations

Urgent dialysis should be considered for patients with severe hyperkalemia and dialysis-dependent renal failure.

Cardiac monitoring is crucial because of the risk of arrhythmia.

References

Gennari FJ: Disorders of potassium homeostasis: hypokalemia and hyperkalemia. *Crit Care Clin* 18:273–288, 2002.

Kamel KS, Wei C: Controversial issues in the treatment of hyperkalaemia. *Nephrol Dial Transplant* 18:2215–2218, 2003.

Kim H, Han S: Therapeutic approach to hyperkalemia. *Nephron* 92(suppl 1):33–40, 2002.

Rastergar A, Soleimani M: Hypokalaemia and hyperkalaemia. *Postgrad Med J* 77:759–764, 2001.

Weiss-Guillet E-M, Takala J, Jakob SM: Diagnosis and management of electrolyte emergencies. *Best Pract Res Clin Endocrinol Metab* 17:623–651, 2003.

Hyponatremia

Hyponatremia is usually secondary to another medical condition causing:

- Volume depletion, which leads to appropriate secretion of antidiuretic hormone (ADH) and resultant hyponatremia; *or*
- Volume overload with ineffective circulating volume, such as cirrhosis, heart failure, or nephrotic syndrome; *or*
- Inappropriate secretion of ADH, most commonly caused by drugs, pulmonary disease, or malignancy. These patients appear clinically euvolemic.

Appropriate admit orders depend on your initial assessment of the patient's volume status and the likely cause of the hyponatremia. ●

These orders are for a patient with hyponatremia in the setting of cirrhosis.

Admit to: Floor

Patients with mild to moderate hyponatremia are typically admitted to the floor. Patients with severe hyponatremia requiring frequent labs or hyponatremia in the setting of significant symptoms (e.g., seizures, obtundation, or hemodynamic instability) require ICU admission.

D iagnosis: Hyponatremia

C ondition: Stable

Many patients with hyponatremia are asymptomatic and clinically stable; hyponatremia requiring ICU admission is life-threatening and status should be critical. **C**

V ital Signs:

Routine
Check orthostatic vital signs
   Orthostatic vital signs can be helpful in assessing volume status, which is the most crucial step in diagnosing and treating hyponatremia. **B**

A llergies: Routine

A ctivity: Up with Assistance

Activity may be ad lib if the patient is without symptoms; hyponatremia may cause weakness, with associated impaired mobility and stability—such patients should be up with assistance only, or at bedrest. Patients with recent seizures attributed to hyponatremia should also be up with assistance only, until severe hyponatremia is corrected. **C**

N ursing

Strict I/O (with Foley catheter if required), daily weights, seizure precautions
   Accurate, ongoing assessment of volume status is paramount in the diagnosis and management of hyponatremia, so strict I/O and daily weights should be done. **C**
   If a patient has had seizure attributed to hyponatremia or sodium is < 120 mEq/L, seizure precautions should be observed. **C**

D iet: 4 g Sodium

Restrict free water to 1.0 L/day

Diet orders should be based on your assessment of the patient's volume status, initial diagnosis, and comorbidities. The patient should be NPO if alterations in mental status due to low sodium preclude safe PO intake.

A low-sodium diet should be prescribed if the patient is clinically volume overloaded or in the setting of congestive heart failure (CHF), cirrhosis, or renal failure.

Free water restriction should be ordered unless hyponatremia is clearly due to volume depletion, which is treated with saline. **C**

IV Fluids: None

Judicious fluid management (administration and withholding) is the mainstay of therapy for hyponatremia. Accurate diagnosis is the first step. Patients who are clinically hypovolemic should be treated with IV fluids for correction. Those who are euvolemic (i.e., syndrome of inappropriate antidiuretic hormone [SIADH]) or hypervolemic should be free water restricted. Initially, free water should be withheld from all hyponatremic patients to avoid exacerbation. **C**

In general, correction should be limited to no more than 8 mEq/L/day to reduce the risk of central pontine myelinolysis. **B**

Fluid Restriction

The recommended free water restriction varies in the literature from 800–1500 mL/day. **C**

Using Intravenous Fluids to Correct Hyponatremia

If patient is severely symptomatic (seizure, severe alteration in mental status), the sodium should be corrected at 1–2 mEq/L/h until symptoms improve or sodium is > 118 mEq/L, in an ICU. 3% hypertonic saline is only appropriate for brief, closely monitored therapy in an ICU (3% = 513 mEq of Na/L). Use hypertonic saline only for the first 3 or 4 hours or until symptoms improve (whichever comes first) and then switch fluids to NS. **C**

Selecting an Initial Fluid Rate

1. Calculate the sodium deficit: (desired Na − actual Na) × total body water (TBW). TBW = weight in kg × (0.5 for women *or* 0.6 for men).
2. Divide the Na deficit by the amount of Na in each liter of your chosen fluid (154 mEq/L for 0.9% NS, 77 mEq/L for 0.45% NS). This translates to the number of liters of fluid necessary to achieve that result.
3. Multiple by 1000 to convert liters to mL.
4. Divide by 24 (hours/day) to provide an hourly infusion rate.

Another useful formula:
Change in serum Na with infusion of 1 L of fluid = infusate Na − serum Na / TBW + 1

Medications:

Hold medications that are believed to be causing or exacerbating hyponatremia

The list of medications that may be associated with hyponatremia is long, but the most commonly implicated include thiazide and loop diuretics, which may cause euvolemic or hypovolemic hyponatremia; NSAIDs; tricyclic antidepressants (TCAs); antiepileptics; and selective serotonin reuptake inhibitors (SSRIs). **B**

Furosemide 20–40 mg IV twice a day (bid) may be used with saline in patients who are euvolemic or hypervolemic when rapid correction is necessary. **B**

Demeclocycline 600–1200 mg/day may be used in patients with chronic SIADH who are unable to avoid symptomatic hyponatremia with fluid restriction alone. **B**

Labs and Diagnostic Studies:

CBC, Chem 10, urine sodium and urine creatinine, serum and urine osmolality

The urine sodium and creatinine and serum and urine sodium are key to diagnosing the cause of hyponatremia. ◉

1. First, measure serum osmolality (low < 265 mOsm/kg water, normal 265–280 mOsm/kg water, high > 280 mOsm/kg water).

    Most patients with hyponatremia will have low osmolality; normal serum osmolality suggests pseudohyponatremia caused by high plasma lipid or proteins levels; high serum osmolality is most often caused by hyperglycemia.

2. Ascertain volume status: Is the patient hypovolemic, euvolemic, or hypervolemic?

3. Check urine sodium (low < 10–20 mEq/24 h) and urine osmolality (low < 100 mOsm/kg water).

Most hypo-osmolar euvolemic patients have SIADH, a diagnosis of exclusion based on the presence of euvolemia associated with elevated urine osmolality (> 100 mOsm/kg water) and normal thyroid function and adrenal axis. SIADH is most often related to medications, chronic illness, and cerebral, pulmonary, or malignant disorders.

Hypo-osmolar hypovolemic patients are losing sodium via the kidneys or elsewhere (distinguish based on urine sodium, which is low if the losses are extrarenal).

Hypo-osmolar hypervolemic patients may have CHF, cirrhosis, nephrotic syndrome, or renal failure (urine sodium is low in states of decreased effective circulating volume [e.g., CHF, cirrhosis, or nephrotic syndrome] but may be high in renal failure).

If volume status is normal and urine osmolality is low (< 100 mOsm/kg water), this suggests excessive fluid intake (beer potomania or psychogenic polydipsia). ◉

Hypothyroidism and adrenal insufficiency can cause hyponatremia—check for them if there is no obvious cause, with thyroid-stimulating hormone (TSH) and AM cortisol or adrenocorticotropic hormone (ACTH) stimulation test. ◉

Discharge Planning:

If medications have been identified as likely culprits and have been discontinued, alternative medications should be considered prior to discharge.

Special Considerations:

When treating hyponatremia, it is critical to avoid correcting the sodium too fast, which can cause central pontine myelinolysis, a severe, irreversible neurologic disorder. For asymptomatic patients, aim for correction of 8 mEq/L/24 h. Patients with severe symptoms initially need to be corrected more quickly, 1–2 mEq/L/h for the first several hours, but labs should be followed very closely to ensure that you do not overshoot. Even for symptomatic patients, serum sodium should not be allowed to rise more than 12 mEq/L over the first 24 hours of treatment. ◉

References

Adrogue HJ: Consequences of inadequate management of hyponatremia. *Am J Nephrol* 25:240–249, 2005.

Adrogue HJ, Madias NE: Hyponatremia. *N Engl J Med* 342:1581–1589, 2000.

Goh KP: Management of hyponatremia. *Am Fam Physician* 69:2387–2394, 2004.

Palmer BF, Gates JR, Lader M: Causes and management of hyponatremia. *Ann Pharmacother* 37:1694–1702, 2003.

Tareen N, Martins D, Nagami G, et al: Sodium disorders in the elderly. *J Natl Med Assoc* 97:217–224, 2005.

Vachharajani TJ, Zaman F, Abreo KD: Hyponatremia in critically ill patients. *J Intensive Care Med* 18:3–8, 2003.

Weiss-Guillet E, Takala J, Jakob SM: Diagnosis and management of electrolyte emergencies. *Best Pract Res Clin Endocrinol Metab* 17:623–651, 2003.

Nephrolithiasis

Patients with nephrolithiasis can often be managed as outpatients but require admission in the event of:

1. Uncontrolled pain
2. Evidence of infection
3. Acute renal insufficiency
4. Inability to tolerate oral fluids or pain medications **C**

Admit to: Floor

Nephrolithiasis can almost always be managed on the floor. An exception would be UTI in the setting of an obstructing stone, which can lead to severe sepsis. A patient with evidence of sepsis should be admitted to the ICU, with prompt imaging and urology consultation.

Diagnosis: Nephrolithiasis

Condition: Stable

Patients with urinary obstruction complicated by obstruction can be critically ill and require urgent decompression. However, most patients with nephrolithiasis are stable.

Vital Signs:

Routine

A llergies: NKDA

A ctivity: Ad Lib

To prevent falls, patients receiving narcotics, especially the elderly, should be cautioned to get up only with assistance.

N ursing:

Strain the urine and save all stones for analysis. If stone has not passed by discharge, send patient home with a strainer

The urine is strained both to document that a stone has passed and to allow analysis of stone composition. More than two-thirds of stones will pass within 1 month of presentation. If a stone does not pass within 1 month, urology referral for intervention is warranted. **©**

Recovered stones should be sent for lab analysis because stone composition will guide further therapy. **©**

D iet: Diet as Tolerated

At least 2 L of fluid per day

Many patients with nephrolithiasis have severe nausea and vomiting and may not be able to take PO.

In the long term, increasing daily urine volume can prevent recurrent stones. A randomized trial of increased fluid intake in 199 patients with their first calcium stone showed a > 50% reduction in the risk of recurrent stones. Patients should be counseled to drink enough water to make urine clear, not yellow. **Ⓐ**

A low-calcium diet is *not* recommended for patients with kidney stones. In a prospective study, patients with the lowest calcium intake had an increased risk of developing recurrent stones. **Ⓑ**

IV Fluids: D5 $\frac{1}{2}$ NS at 100 mL/h

Overhydration should be avoided because urine flow and ureteral distention will increase and worsen pain. **C**

Medications:

Ketorolac 25 mg IV × 1 now. May repeat q 6 hours prn pain for 24 hours

Morphine sulfate 2–5 mg IV q 3 hours prn pain not relieved by ketorolac

NSAIDs, particularly when administered parenterally, are at least as effective as narcotics in relieving the often severe pain of acute renal colic and are less likely to cause nausea. **A**

However, NSAIDs should be *avoided* in patients with renal insufficiency, CHF, a single or transplanted kidney, or volume depletion because the risk of renal insufficiency is increased.

Labs and Diagnostic Studies:

CBC, Chem 7, serum calcium, UA and culture
Noncontrast helical CT of the abdomen and pelvis ("CT-KUB")
Stone composition analysis if stone is recovered

UA demonstrates hematuria in 80–90% of patients presenting with nephrolithiasis. The presence of hematuria supports a diagnosis of nephrolithiasis but is not specific. Further imaging studies are usually performed to confirm the diagnosis.

Noncontrast helical CT has become the initial diagnostic procedure of choice at most hospitals because it has high sensitivity, has high specificity, and can be performed rapidly. **A**

Ultrasound is less sensitive and specific than CT but is a reasonable first test in pregnant patients or when CT is not available. **A**

Stone composition is helpful in guiding further therapy, so recovered stones should be sent for analysis. ◉

Discharge Planning:

Patients may be discharged when the stone has passed and symptoms have resolved. Patients with persistent obstruction may be discharged if symptoms are controlled on oral medications, provided renal function is normal and there is no evidence of infection. ◉

Special Considerations:

Urgent urology consultation should be requested in patients with stones and evidence of infection, acute renal insufficiency, intractable pain or vomiting, or obstruction of a solitary or transplanted kidney. ◉

Less urgent consultation should be obtained for stones larger than 1 cm, which are unlikely to pass spontaneously, and stones that have not passed after 1 month of watchful waiting. ◉

Reference

Teichman JM: Acute renal colic from ureteral calculus. *N Engl J Med* 350:684–693, 2004.

Prevention of Contrast Nephropathy

Contrast nephropathy is a typically mild, reversible form of nonoliguric renal failure that develops soon after the administration of IV contrast for a CT scan or angiogram.

Risk factors for more severe renal failure, which may even require hemodialysis, include:

- Chronic renal insufficiency, with GFR < 60 mL/min or creatinine > 1.5 mg/dL
- Diabetic nephropathy
- Decompensated heart failure
- Volume depletion
- Hypoalbuminemia
- Multiple myeloma

Specific measures to prevent contrast nephropathy should be considered for patients with these risk factors.

These orders are for a 71-year-old woman with diabetes, proteinuria, and a creatinine of 1.6 mg/dL admitted with increasing chest pain for cardiac catheterization in the morning.

A dmit to: Telemetry Floor

The level of care is dictated by the underlying condition requiring imaging.

D iagnosis: Prevention of Contrast Nephropathy

C ondition: Stable

V ital Signs:

Every 4 hours, with oxygen saturation
Call house officer (HO) for decreasing O_2 saturation, HR > 110 bpm, SBP > 160 mmHg

Sodium bicarbonate, which may be used to prevent contrast nephropathy, can cause volume overload and hypertension. Patients should be monitored carefully.

A llergies: NKDA

A ctivity: As Tolerated

N ursing:

Strict I/Os; daily weights including weight on admission

D iet: NPO for Planned Procedure in the Morning

IV Fluids:

Sodium bicarbonate 150 mEq/L at 3 mL/kg/h IV for 1 hour prior to, followed by 1 mL/kg/h IV during contrast exposure and for 6 hours thereafter

A single randomized trial has shown bicarbonate to be effective in preventing contrast nephropathy in at-risk patients. **Ⓐ**

A sodium bicarbonate 150 mEq/L solution can be prepared by mixing three 50-mEq ampules of sodium bicarbonate in 1 L of D5W.

Volume depletion should be corrected prior to contrast administration and carefully avoided for 2 days after contrast.

M edications:

N-acetylcysteine 600 mg PO bid on the day prior to and day of contrast administration
Hold **hydrochlorothiazide until hospital discharge**
Atenolol 100 mg PO qd
Atorvastatin 40 mg PO qd
Aspirin (ASA) 325 mg PO qd
Insulin glargine 20 units SQ tonight

Multiple randomized trials of N-acetylcysteine have shown inconsistent results in preventing contrast nephropathy. Some have shown marked benefit, whereas others have shown no benefit. Nevertheless, it is inexpensive and has few side effects and is a reasonable therapy for patients at increased risk. **Ⓑ**

N-acetylcysteine smells and tastes of rotten eggs. Some have found that mixing it in a cola drink makes it more tolerable.

Because volume depletion increases the risk of nephropathy, consider holding diuretics around the time of contrast administration. ☉

NSAIDs should also be held, if possible, around the time of contrast administration. ☉

L abs and Diagnostic Studies:

Daily Chem 7

The serum creatinine typically begins to rise soon after contrast administration. If the creatinine is stable 48 hours later, the subsequent development of nephropathy is unlikely.

D ischarge Planning:

Discharge planning is guided by the underlying diagnosis.

Patients at high risk for contrast nephropathy should receive IV sodium bicarbonate for 6 hours after contrast but can then be discharged home to continue oral hydration if otherwise stable.

Consider checking a serum creatinine 48 hours following contrast in high-risk patients prior to allowing them to resume metformin or nephrotoxic medications.

References

Aspelin P, Aubry P, Fransson SG, et al: Nephrotoxic effects in high risk patients undergoing angiography. *N Engl J Med* 348:491–499, 2003.

Birck R, Krzossok S, Markowetz F, et al: Acetylcysteine for prevention of contrast nephropathy: Meta-analysis. *Lancet* 362:598–603, 2003.

Fishbane S, Purham JH, Marzo K, et al: N-acetylcysteine in the prevention of radiocontrast-induced nephropathy. *J Am Soc Nephrol* 15:251–260, 2004.

Marenzi G, Bartorelli A: Recent advances in the prevention of radiocontrast-induced nephropathy. *Curr Opin Crit Care* 10:505–509, 2004.

Merten GJ, Burgess WP, Gray LV, et al: Prevention of contrast-induced nephropathy with sodium bicarbonate: A randomized controlled trial. *JAMA* 291:2328–2334, 2004.

Tepel M, Aspelin P, Lameire N: Contrast induced nephropathy: A clinical and evidence based approach. *Circulation* 113:1799–1806, 2006.

Deep Vein Thrombosis and Pulmonary Embolism

Deep vein thrombosis (DVT) and pulmonary embolism (PE) (collectively called *venous thromboembolism* [VTE]) are common reasons for hospital admission. Although many patients present with either leg symptoms leading to a diagnosis of DVT or pulmonary symptoms leading to a diagnosis of PE, there is overlap. Patients with DVT but no pulmonary symptoms are frequently found to have pulmonary emboli if tested, and those with PE are presumed to have had DVT as the source of emboli. Therefore, the two clinical entities are felt to be manifestations of the same disease, and basic therapy is the same.

Carefully selected patients with DVT and PE can be managed primarily at home with low-molecular-weight heparin (LMWH) and warfarin anticoagulation. These patients may receive initial education and coordination of care in the emergency department (ED) or in an observation unit. The minimal requirements for early outpatient treatment are:

- A physician responsible for ongoing care
- Stable patient with normal vital signs and without significant underlying cardiopulmonary disease
- Low bleeding risk
- Practical system for administration and monitoring of LMWH and warfarin
- Patient education about symptoms of recurrent VTE and bleeding complications

---

Ⓐ Recommendation based on consistent and good quality patient-oriented evidence. Ⓑ Recommendation based on inconsistent or limited quality patient-oriented evidence. Ⓒ Recommendation based on usual practice, consensus, opinion, disease-oriented evidence, or case series for studies of diagnosis, treatment, and prevention of screening.

The Geneva scoring system for identifying low-risk patients with PE has been developed and validated retrospectively. It may be used to identify patients with PE who are stable for early discharge. ❸

These orders are for a 78-year-old woman with a recent knee arthroplasty and 4 days of shortness of breath, with a left upper lobe (LUL) PE demonstrated on spiral CT.

A dmit to: Floor

Patients with PE and shock, clinical or echocardiographic evidence of right ventricular dysfunction without shock, and severe underlying cardiopulmonary disease should be admitted to the ICU. Other patients may be admitted to the floor. ❸

D iagnosis: Deep Vein Thrombosis and Pulmonary Embolism

C ondition: Guarded

The mortality of PE with shock is 25–50%, and with right ventricular dysfunction, 10–20%. The condition of such patients is critical.

Patients with no shock or right ventricular dysfunction have much lower mortality, < 2%.

V ital Signs:

Every 2 hours × 4, then q 4 hours
Call for HR > 100 bpm or SBP < 100 mmHg

Otherwise healthy patients with large pulmonary emboli may appear deceptively well at presentation but develop shock hours later. Frequent vital signs are initially warranted. ❸

A llergies: NKDA

Activity: Up with Assistance, Fall Precautions

There is no evidence that bedrest reduces the risk of recurrent PE in clinically stable patients with VTE. However, these patients should be cautious when ambulating because a fall is more likely to cause significant injury due to anticoagulation. ☉

Nursing:

Oxygen by nasal cannula to maintain O_2 saturation > 92%
No IM injections

IM injections should be avoided in anticoagulated or thrombocytopenic patients to avoid hematoma formation. ☉

Diet: General

A nutritionist or pharmacist should educate the patient about vitamin K in the diet, in anticipation of long-term treatment with warfarin.

Fluids: None

Maintenance IV fluids are not necessary if the patient is able to eat and drink. Hypotensive patients should receive aggressive volume resuscitation, in addition to other therapy.

Medications:

Enoxaparin 70 mg (1 mg/k) SQ q 12 hours
Warfarin 5 mg PO tonight. Check warfarin dose qd
Acetaminophen 650 mg PO q 6 hours prn pain
Oxycodone 5–10 mg PO q 6 hours prn pain

LMWH, such as enoxaparin, has predictable dose requirements and requires less monitoring than unfractionated heparin. Cost-effectiveness analyses show overall cost savings with LMWH as initial therapy for VTE. Critically ill patients, who may require thrombolysis or invasive procedures, should be treated with unfractionated heparin rather than LMWH, which cannot be rapidly reversed. LMWH is also contraindicated in renal insufficiency and severe obesity. **Ⓐ**

If unfractionated heparin is used, it should be given as an initial bolus of 80 mg/kg, then an infusion of 18 mg/kg. A standardized dose adjustment protocol is a safe and effective way of maintaining the partial thromboplastin time (PTT) in the therapeutic range. **Ⓐ**

Warfarin can be started on the same day. A 5-mg loading dose may be less likely to cause early overanticoagulation than a 10-mg loading dose. Either IV heparin or LMWH should be continued for at least 5 days and until the international normalized ratio (INR) is therapeutic on 2 consecutive days. **Ⓑ**

Peripheral pulmonary emboli may cause pleuritic chest pain, requiring analgesics. NSAIDs should be avoided, if possible, in anticoagulated patients. **Ⓒ**

Labs and Diagnostic Studies:

Chem 7, liver function tests (LFTs), calcium, urinalysis (UA), ECG on admit
Complete blood count (CBC) with platelets qd
INR qd

Undiagnosed malignancy may present with VTE Basic laboratory tests should be performed on admission, as well as a full physical exam and any age-appropriate cancer screening that has not recently been done. **Ⓑ**

Nephrotic syndrome may present with VTE due to loss of anticoagulant proteins in the urine. A UA should be performed to detect significant proteinuria. **Ⓒ**

ECG changes are common in PE, but none are sensitive or specific for the diagnosis. An ECG can provide clues to right ventricular strain, which may alter therapy. **Ⓒ**

Heparin-induced thrombocytopenia (HIT) occurs in 0.3–3% of patients treated with unfractionated heparin for more than 4 days. The risk of HIT is lower in patients treated with LMWH. CBC with platelet count should be checked daily for hospitalized patients. ❸

INR should be checked daily in inpatients to adjust warfarin dose. ❸

PTT should be checked daily and 6 hours after every dose change for patients on unfractionated heparin, but those treated with enoxaparin do not require routine monitoring of the PTT. ❹

Discharge Planning:

Patient and family education about anticoagulation should be started as soon after admission as possible and should cover side effects, administration of LMWH, and monitoring. If the patient has no contraindications to LMWH and has normal vital signs, he or she may be discharged on LMWH and warfarin as soon as education is completed and close follow-up is arranged.

Either a nutritionist or pharmacist should also provide teaching about vitamin K in the diet. ❻

Follow-up for an INR should be schedule in an anticoagulation clinic or the patient's primary care clinic 2 days postdischarge. Close follow-up of anticoagulation is crucial in the early stages of management—anticoagulation clinics have been shown to decrease the rate of complications of anticoagulation. ❹

Provide a prescription for 30-mmHg graduated compression stockings at discharge. In patients with symptomatic DVT, support hose halved the incidence of postphlebitic syndrome at 2 years follow-up. ❹

Special Considerations:

Thrombolysis is typically recommended for patients with massive PE, defined as PE with hemodynamic instability, who are not at major risk for bleeding. **B**

There is no consensus on the use of thrombolysis for submassive PE, defined as clinical or echocardiographic evidence of right ventricular strain. Pulmonary/critical care consultation is recommended when thrombolysis is being considered for this indication.

If anticoagulation is contraindicated in acute VTE, an inferior vena caval filter should be placed. **C**

References

Buller HR, Agnelli G, Hull RD, et al: Antithrombotic therapy for venous thromboembolic disease. *Chest* 126:401S–428S, 2004.

Konstantinides S, Geibel A, Heusel G, et al: Heparin plus alteplase compared withheparin alone for submassive pulmonary embolism. *N Engl J Med* 347:1143–1150, 2002.

Nendaz MR, Bandelier P, Aujesky D, et al: Validation of a risk score identifying patients with acute pulmonary embolism, who are at low risk of clinical adverse outcome. *Thromb Haemost* 91:1232–1236, 2004.

Community-Acquired Pneumonia in Immunocompetent Adults

Community-acquired pneumonia (CAP) is a very common reason for ED evaluation and hospital admission.

The initial site of care should be determined with a three-step process:

1. Assess for conditions that would compromise the safety of home care; for example, chronic hypoxia or inability to take oral medications.

2. Calculate the PORT Severity Index (PSI), which assigns points for patient age, comorbidity and clinical and laboratory factors on admission to assess severity of illness (*see* Table 1 for scoring system).

3. Use clinical judgment in the decision to treat as an outpatient. Substance abuse, homelessness, psychiatric illness, and poor social support, among other factors, may necessitate inpatient care. Clinical judgment supersedes the PSI score.

A dmit to: Floor

The PSI can help triage patients to the appropriate site of initial care: **A**

- Class I and Class II patients can usually be treated as outpatients (0.6% 30-day mortality).
- Class III patients (0.9–2.8% mortality) can be treated at home if stable after a brief period of observation.
- Patients in Class IV (~9% mortality) and Class V severity (27% mortality) should be admitted. Patients in risk Class V should be admitted to the ICU. **A**

D iagnosis: Community-Acquired Pneumonia in an Immunocompetent Adult

C ondition: Stable

V ital Signs: Routine

Admission vital signs must include an assessment of oxygenation.

Table 1 Point Scoring System for Hospital Admission (Modified from Pneumonia Patient Outcomes Research Team [PORT], modified from Fine 1997): *Pneumonia Severity Index Score*

		Points
Demographics		
	Age–men	Age in years
	Age–women	Age in years–10
	Nursing home residence	+ 10
Comorbidity		
	Malignancy	+ 30
	Liver disease	+ 20
	Congestive heart failure	+ 10
	Cerebrovascular disease	+ 10
	Renal disease	+ 10
Physical examination findings		
	Altered mental status	+ 20
	Respiratory rate $\geq$ 30 per minute	+ 20
	Systolic blood pressure < 90 mmHg	+ 10
	Temperature < 35°C or $\geq$ 40°C	+ 15
	Heart rate $\geq$ 125 beats per minute	+ 10
Laboratory/radiographic findings		
	Arterial pH < 7.35	+ 30
	Blood urea nitrogen $\geq$ 30 mg/dL	+ 20
	Sodium < 130 mmol/L	+ 20
	Glucose $\geq$ 250 mg/dL	+ 10
	Hematocrit < 30%	+ 10

Continued

Table 1 Point Scoring System for Hospital Admission (Modified from Pneumonia Patient Outcomes Research Team [PORT], modified from Fine 1997):

Pneumonia Severity Index Score—Cont'd

PaO2 < 60 mmHg	+ 10
Pleural effusion	+ 10

Recommendations:
Class I and II: consider outpatient therapy
Class III: consider brief inpatient observation
Class IV and V: admit

Mortality Risk:
< 70 points – Class II: 0.6–0.7%
71–90 points – Class III: 0.9–2.8%
91–130 points – Class IV: 8.2–9.3%
> 130 points – Class V: 27–31%

A llergies: NKDA

A ctivity: Activity as Tolerated

Most patients sick enough to be admitted to the hospital for pneumonia will not be able to ambulate without oxygen. Activity should be encouraged only as tolerated.

N ursing:

Supplemental oxygen via nasal cannula to maintain O_2 saturation > 91%

In patients without preexisting obstructive lung disease, sufficient oxygen to maintain O_2 saturation > 91% should be given. Patients with severe obstructive lung disease, particularly those with a history of carbon dioxide retention, may rely on the hypoxic drive to drive respiration. In these patients, O_2 saturation should be maintained of 88–91%. ⦿

D iet: Regular

Patients with suspected aspiration pneumonia should be NPO until swallowing is evaluated, either by a speech pathologist or with a barium pharyngogram, to avoid recurrent aspiration. ⦿

IV Fluids: D5 $\frac{1}{2}$ Normal Saline (NS) at 100 mL/h

Patients not able to take PO fluids require maintenance IV fluids. If the patient is volume depleted (dry mucous membranes, flat neck veins, orthostatic), volume resuscitate with NS. If the patient is able to tolerate oral intake, maintenance IV fluids are not necessary. ⦿

Medications:

Ceftriaxone 1 g IV q 24 hours—administer ASAP
Azithromycin 500 mg IV q 24 hours—administer ASAP
Acetaminophen 650 mg PO q 6 hours prn pain or fever
Oxycodone 5–10 mg PO q 6 hours prn pleuritic chest pain not
  relieved by acetaminophen
Heparin 5000 units SQ q 8 hours

Empiric antibiotics should be administered within 4 hours of presentation to the ED. Early antibiotic administration improves mortality and hospital length of stay. Time to antibiotic administration is also a Joint Committee on Accreditation of Health Care Organizations (JCAHO) core measure of hospital quality. **Ⓐ**

Empiric antibiotic regimens for patients admitted to the general medicine ward should include coverage for atypical organisms and should avoid classes of drugs that have been prescribed in the past 3 months. **Ⓑ**

Recommended empiric regimens include:

- Ceftriaxone 1 g IV every 24 hours *and* azithromycin 500 mg IV/PO every 24 hours, *or*
- Moxifloxacin 400 mg *or* levofloxacin 500–750 mg IV/PO every 24 hours

If aspiration is suspected, anaerobes should be covered. Suggested regimens include:

- Ampicillin/sulbactam 1.5 g IV q 6 hours
- For penicillin-allergic patients: clindamycin 600 mg IV every 8 hours and levofloxacin 500 mg IV/PO q 24 hours, *or* Moxifloxacin 400 mg IV/PO q 24 hours

Patients admitted to the ICU are more likely to have resistant pathogens, including *Legionella,* and are covered more broadly. Suggested regimens include:

- Ceftriaxone 1 g IV every 24 hours *and* either azithromycin or a respiratory fluoroquinolone (levofloxacin or moxifloxacin)
- If *Pseudomonas* is suspected, an antipseudomonal antibiotic, such as piperacillin/tazobactam, imipenem, meropenem, or cefepime, *plus* either azithromycin or a respiratory fluoroquinolone
- If methicillin-resistant *Staphylococcus aureus* (MRSA) is suspected based on history or sputum Gram stain, consider vancomycin pending culture results

Antibiotic therapy should be tailored as soon as the causative organism is identified.

Timely transition to oral antibiotics has been shown to decrease hospital length of stay. Consider switching to oral therapy if the patient is clinically improving with decreasing cough/dyspnea, has been afebrile for 16 hours, is tolerating oral intake, and has normal vital signs (HR < 100 bpm, BP > 90 mmHg). ❸

Most pneumonia patients sick enough to be admitted to the hospital are nonambulatory and should be given DVT prophylaxis.

Labs and Diagnostic Studies:

Chem 7, CBC with differential
Blood cultures × 2, sputum Gram stain and culture prior to antibiotics
Arterial blood gas (ABG)
Posteroanterior (PA) and lateral chest x-ray (CXR) on admit

Admission studies can help with assessment of severity of illness and guide therapy. Assessment of renal function is critical to appropriately dose drugs.

A low white blood count (WBC) ($< 4000/mm^3$) is associated with a poor prognosis in patients with pneumonia. ❸

Sputum Gram stain and culture is controversial. If a predominant organism is identified by Gram stain or culture, therapy can be tailored to that organism. However, this is not a common finding, and sputum culture has never been shown to improve outcomes of patients admitted with pneumonia.

Blood cultures are positive in ~10% of patients with CAP. If positive, blood cultures identify high-risk patients and may also help to tailor therapy. In one study, the performance of blood cultures within 24 hours of arrival was associated with a 10% reduction in 30-day mortality, presumably because positive cultures pinpointed a subgroup of patients at higher risk who could be treated more aggressively. A targeted approach to performance of blood cultures has been shown to identify 88–89% of bacteremic patients and to reduce the number of cultures done by 38%. However, performance of blood cultures in patients admitted with CAP is a JCAHO core measure of hospital quality, so many hospitals prefer a policy of routine blood cultures at the time of admission, prior to antibiotic administration. **ⓒ**

ABG should be performed if O_2 saturation is less than 91% on room air or if respiratory distress is present. PaO_2 < 60 mmHg is associated with worse prognosis.

Elderly patients, those with comorbid pulmonary disease, or those admitted to the ICU may also be evaluated for *Legionella* with a urinary antigen test. The recommended macrolide or quinolone will cover *Legionella*, however.

A CXR is recommended in all cases of suspected CAP, both to establish diagnosis and to assess for complications such as parapneumonic effusion. **ⓒ**

A normal CXR, however, does not rule out CAP, particularly if pretest probability is high. Up to one-third of CAP cases have equivocal findings on CXR; 15–30% of those with a "negative" CXR have findings suggestive of pneumonia on CT. Consider chest CT if there is no response to initial therapy or if there is evidence of a large or loculated pleural effusion on plain film. **C**

Discharge Planning:

A patient with CAP can usually be safely discharged if he or she has normal vital signs and normal mental status, is able to tolerate oral antibiotic therapy/oral intake, and has a safe environment to go to. Objective criteria for safety of discharge have been identified, including: HR < 100 bpm, SBP > 90 mmHg, RR ≤ 24 breaths/minute, O_2 saturation ≥ 90%, temperature ≤ 37.8°C, ability to tolerate oral intake, and normal mental status. Patients should remain hospitalized until all but one of these criteria are present for at least 24 hours. **B**

References

Fine MJ, Auble TE, Yealy DM, et al: A prediction rule to identify low risk patients with community acquired pneumonia. *N Engl J Med* 336:243–250, 1997.

Halm EA, Lee C, Chassin MR: Instability on hospital discharge and the risk of adverse outcomes in patients with pneumonia. *Arch Intern Med* 162:1278–1284, 2002.

Mandell LA, Bartlett JG, Dowell SF, et al: IDSA guidelines: Update of practice guidelines for the management of community acquired pneumonia in immunocompetent adults. *Clin Infect Dis* 37:1405–1433, 2003.

Metlay JP, Fine MJ: Testing strategies in the initial management of patients with community acquired pneumonia. *Ann Intern Med* 138:109–118, 2003.

Chronic Obstructive Pulmonary Disease Exacerbation

Patients with chronic obstructive pulmonary disease (COPD) exacerbation should be admitted if they have:

- Worsening hypoxemia
- Worsening hypercarbia
- Altered mentation
- Failure to respond to outpatient medications
- Inability to walk between rooms or to eat or to sleep due to dyspnea
- High-risk comorbid condition (pulmonary or nonpulmonary), including pneumonia, cardiac arrhythmia, congestive heart failure, diabetes mellitus, or renal or liver failure
- Inability to care for self

A dmit to: ICU

ICU admission is typically recommended for patients with:

- Confusion, lethargy, or respiratory muscle fatigue
- Worsening hypoxemia despite supplemental O_2
- Worsening acidosis or pH < 7.3
- Need for mechanical ventilation
- Inadequate response to ED therapies

More stable patients can be admitted to the floor.

D iagnosis: COPD

C ondition: Critical

Clinical status of floor patients may be stable or guarded.

V ital Signs: ICU Routine

A llergies: Routine

A ctivity: As Tolerated

Seriously ill patients are unlikely to be able to get out of bed independently.

N ursing:

O_2 to maintain O_2 saturation of 89–91%

Oxygen should be titrated to balance two goals: preventing tissue hypoxia while avoiding CO_2 retention. An O_2 saturation of 90% is a "happy medium" because there is little benefit to each percent saturation above 90% (which equates to 60 mmHg), yet the risk of retention increases. ◐

D iet: Regular

IV Fluids: None Needed If Patient Able to Take PO

M edications:

Methylprednisolone 125 mg IV now, then 30 mg IV q 6 hours
Albuterol nebulizer q 4 hours
Ipratropium nebulizer q 4 hours
Albuterol nebulizer q 1 hour prn wheezing or shortness of breath (SOB)
Trimethoprim-sulfamethoxazole (TMP-SMX) 1 double-strength tablet PO bid
Nicotine patch 21 mg applied qd

Corticosteroids are prescribed for almost all patients admitted with COPD exacerbation.

The optimal dose and route of administration have not, however, been well studied. Most hospitalized patients, especially those with the most severe obstruction, are treated initially with IV methylprednisolone. However, once oral medications can be reliably taken and obstruction improves, you can transition to oral prednisone with a typical starting dose of 60 mg PO qd. In severe exacerbations, the prednisone should be tapered slowly. **C**

Aggressive bronchodilator therapy should be ordered on a scheduled basis as well as prn. **A**

Ipratropium nebulizers may provide additional bronchodilation and should be used with albuterol. **A**

Not all exacerbations require antibiotic therapy. Consider antibiotics for patients with:

- Signs or symptoms of infection, including a change in sputum
- Forced expiratory volume in 1 second (FEV_1) < 35% predicted
- > 60 years old

Patients with nonpurulent sputum may improve without antibiotics.

Initial antibiotics could be chosen based on the suspected underlying infection: CAP (ceftriaxone and azithromycin) or acute on chronic bronchitis (doxycycline, amoxicillin/clavulanate, TMP-SMX, fluoroquinolone). **B**

Strongly encourage smoking cessation. Offer assistance while hospitalized, including a nicotine patch and additional resources for abstinence postdischarge. **A**

Labs and Diagnostic Studies:

Admit labs: ABG, CBC, Chem 7
Sputum culture
CXR
ECG

ABG should be checked for all patients with severe symptoms and all patients with altered mental status or sedation, which may be due to hypercarbia. **Ⓒ**

CBC should be done to assess for infection. **Ⓒ**

Sputum and blood cultures are indicated to guide antibiotic choices if infection is suspected. **Ⓒ**

Discharge Planning:

There are several important considerations in planning for discharge of a patient with COPD.

Assessing Need for Home Oxygen

Oxygen improves survival in patients with chronic hypoxia and COPD. Medicare guidelines for home oxygen require an O_2 saturation of $< 88\%$ on room air or a $PaO_2 < 55$ mmHg. Patients with PaO_2 of 55–59 mmHg who have associated pulmonary hypertension, cor pulmonale, erythrocytosis, edema, or altered mental status should also receive home oxygen. **Ⓐ**

If O_2 saturation is $> 88\%$ at rest, measure the O_2 saturation with ambulation. If it falls to $< 88\%$, the patient will also qualify for home O_2. A patient whose HR increases dramatically with mild exertion may also benefit from oxygen use, but insurance coverage in this situation is less certain. **Ⓒ**

Medications

Provide education on the correct use and side effects of medications for COPD. **Ⓒ**

Provide aerosolizing chamber for metered dose inhalers (MDIs) and instruct in their use. **Ⓐ**

Patient Education

Reiterate the importance of smoking cessation. Smoking cessation reduces the rate of decline in lung function in COPD by 50% and is more effective than any medical therapy in improving long-term outcomes. **Ⓐ**

Review indications for calling or returning for follow-up sooner than planned.

Follow-Up

Close outpatient follow-up can decrease the likelihood of readmission.

Consider pulmonary consultation for patients with:

- Age of onset < 40 years
- ≥ 2 episodes/year despite adequate therapy
- Rapidly worsening disease
- Severe disease (FEV_1 < 50%)
- Need for home O_2
- Consideration of need for lung volume reduction surgery

Special Considerations:

Noninvasive Positive Pressure Ventilation (NPPV)

NPPV is delivered by face or nose mask and provides ventilatory support without endotracheal intubation. Continuous positive airway pressure (CPAP) delivers continuous pressure to help maintain an open airway and is most useful in obstructive sleep apnea and hypoxemic respiratory failure.

Biphasic positive airway pressure (BiPAP) delivers two different levels of positive pressure: a higher level during inspiration and a lower level during expiration, to allow more effective exhalation. BiPAP can be very effective in COPD exacerbations, reducing the need for intubation, length of stay, and even mortality. **Ⓐ**

Patients with persistent breathlessness or respiratory acidosis (pH < 7.36) despite appropriate initial therapy can be treated with NPPV. They must be monitored closely in a step-down unit or an ICU. **Ⓒ**

NPPV is contraindicated with: **Ⓒ**

- Respiratory arrest
- Cardiovascular instability (hypotension, arrhythmias, myocardial infarction)
- Impaired mental status, somnolence, or inability to cooperate
- Copious and/or viscous secretions with high aspiration risk
- Recent facial or gastroesophageal surgery
- Craniofacial trauma and/or fixed nasopharyngeal abnormality
- Facial burns
- Extreme obesity

References

Lightowler JV, Wedzicha JA, Elliot M, Ram SF: Non invasive positive pressure ventilation to treat respiratory failure resulting from exacerbations of chronic obstructive pulmonary disease: Cochrane systematic review and meta-analysis. *BMJ* 326:185–189, 2003.

pier.acponline.org/physicians/diseases/d153/d153.html.

www.thoracic.org/COPD/exacerbation.asp.

Asthma Exacerbation

Patients with asthma may improve with initial ED therapy, allowing discharge.

Risk factors for relapse after initial improvement should be considered in triage. The following factors increase risk and should significantly lower the threshold for admission: **❸**

- Prior intubation
- History of labile asthma
- Frequent hospitalizations

- ED visit in the past 12 months for asthma
- Low adherence to inhaled steroids

Other factors that may influence the severity of the exacerbation may include depression, substance abuse, personality disorders, unemployment, or recent bereavement. ❸

A dmit to: ICU

ICU admission is recommended in the following situations: ❸

- Status asthmaticus
- Peak flow rates that are < 30% predicted, that improve < 10% post-treatment, or that fluctuate wildly are associated with a higher risk of death.
- Signs of impending respiratory failure (altered mentation, worsening fatigue, $pCO_2 > 42$ mmHg) (intubation should be considered early if these patients do not respond quickly to therapy)

More stable patients can be admitted to the floor.

D iagnosis: Asthma Exacerbation

C ondition: Critical

Patients admitted to the floor may be in stable or guarded condition.

V ital Signs:

ICU routine, including continuous O_2 saturation monitoring
Tachycardia may result from beta agonist treatments.

Remember that O_2 saturation may be falsely reassuring in patients with asthma, who may maintain a fairly normal O_2 saturation despite severe airway obstruction and rising CO_2.

If you are concerned about the possibility of respiratory failure, do a blood gas even if the saturation is normal.

Pulsus paradoxus (a drop in SBP of 10 mmHg or more with inspiration) is seen in about 60% of patients with severe airflow obstruction. This exam maneuver is typically performed by the patient's physician rather than by the nurse.

Allergies: Avoid Aspirin (ASA)

Up to 10% of patients with asthma may be sensitive to aspirin

Activity: As Tolerated

Nursing:

Check peak expiratory flow qd and educate patient in performing at home

O_2 to maintain saturation > 90%

Peak expiratory flow can be checked in almost any location in the hospital using a small, portable flow meter and is helpful in following response to therapy. Check peak flow 60–90 minutes after initiation of therapy and after the third dose of therapy. Follow daily peak flow; educate patient in its use and self-charting, and encourage participation with meter. ◉

O_2 saturation should be maintained > 95% in pregnant patients and in those with heart disease. ◉

Remember, do not be falsely reassured by a normal O_2 saturation if the patient appears to be developing respiratory failure.

Diet: Regular

IV Fluids: None Needed If Patient Able to Take PO

Aggressive hydration has not been found to be helpful in adult patients presenting with asthma. ◉

Medications:

Methylprednisolone 125 mg IV now
Prednisone 60 mg PO qd
Albuterol nebulizer q 4 hours
Ipratropium nebulizer q 4 hours
Albuterol nebulizer q 1 hour prn wheezing or SOB
Nicotine patch 14 mg applied qd
Avoid sedatives

Corticosteroid therapy is warranted in moderate to severe attacks and should be given in the ED. Steroids should also be considered in patients who do not respond to bronchodilator therapy. **B**

Oral steroids are equivalent in efficacy to IV steroids in asthma and may be preferable because they are noninvasive. **C** If the patient can take oral medications and the obstruction is improving, you can transition to oral prednisone with a typical starting dose of 60 mg PO daily. In severe exacerbations, the prednisone should be tapered slowly. **C**

High-dose MDIs are as effective as nebulizers when used correctly in a supervised setting. **A**

Ipratropium may provide bronchodilator effect in addition to that of beta agonists. **B**

Methylxanthines, including theophylline and aminophylline, have traditionally been used to treat acute asthma exacerbations but do not clearly provide added benefit. Use of these medications is controversial.

Smoking cessation should be strongly recommended to all patients admitted with asthma. Use of a nicotine patch may help nicotine withdrawal symptoms.

Sedative medications should be avoided because they may decrease respiratory drive and precipitate intubation. **C**

Antibiotics should only be prescribed if there is evidence of infection. **C**

In adult patients, mucolytics have *not* been shown to be helpful.

Labs and Diagnostic Studies:

Admit labs: ABG, CBC, Chem 7, CXR, sputum culture, blood cultures

Daily labs: CBC, chemistry panel

ABG should be checked in all patients with severe symptoms, a peak flow < 30% predicted after treatment, or clinically suspected hypoventilation (altered mental status, accessory muscle use, paradoxical inspiration). Note that a normal pCO_2 may be misleading because during an exacerbation, patients typically have a heightened respiratory drive and should be "blowing off" CO_2. A "normal" pCO_2 of 43 mmHg may mean an asthma patient is well on the way to respiratory failure. ☯

CXR should be performed if there is suspicion of infection, including almost all patients admitted with asthma. CXR may also show complications of the asthma exacerbation, including pneumothorax or pneumomediastinum. ☯

Sputum and blood cultures should be performed in patients diagnosed with pneumonia. ☯

A theophyline level should be checked if the patient is taking it at home because toxicity can lead to an exacerbation. ☯

A chemistry panel should be done daily to monitor for hypokalemia due to beta agonists or corticosteroids and hyponatremia due to pulmonary disease–induced increased antidiuretic hormone (ADH) secretion. The white blood count may be increased by corticosteroids or stress demargination. ☯

ECG should be performed in patients > 50 years or with coexistent heart disease or COPD. *Note:* You may see signs of right heart strain (S1Q3T3) that reverse with treatment of the exacerbation. ☯

Discharge Planning:

Medications

Ensure adequate medications are prescribed. Educate the patient regarding use and side effects. **C**

Consider low-dose inhaled steroid for chronic therapy in patients with mild to moderate persistent asthma. **A**

Provide aerosolizing chamber for MDIs and instruct on itd use. **A**

Patient Education

Provide peak flow monitor, educate regarding its use, and encourage recording the best of three each AM and PM. **C**

Educate each patient on simple facts of asthma, environmental triggers, medications, and importance of self-monitoring. **A**

Consider referral to formal outpatient asthma education course. **C**

Refer smokers for smoking cessation counseling and strongly reinforce the need to quit. **C**

Follow-Up

Arrange follow-up appointment (best if within 7 days). Refer to an asthma specialist if admit was for a life-threatening episode or if the patient has a history of multiple hospitalizations for asthma. **B**

Develop action plan with patient for recurrence or worsening of symptoms. **C**

Special Considerations:

Watch for "danger signs" of impending respiratory failure: altered mental status, diaphoresis, accessory muscle use, and paradoxic respirations.

Consider respiratory therapy consultation for evaluation and assistance with management. **C**

Chest physiotherapy is unlikely to be helpful and may cause added stress. ☯

References

ACP/PIER: Asthma: pier.acponline.org/physicians/diseases/d146/d146.html.

Expert Panel Report 2: Guidelines for the Diagnosis and Management of Asthma. The National Asthma Education and Prevention Program of the National Heart, Lung, and Blood Institute, National Institutes of Health. USDHHS, Public Health Service. NIH publication no. 97–4051. April 1997.

Diabetes Management

Although few patients are admitted with a primary diagnosis of diabetes, diabetics are frequently hospitalized with other illnesses. Hyperglycemia is associated with worse outcomes in acute myocardial infarction (MI), stroke, and general medical patients. It impairs the response to infection and causes osmotic diuresis and nausea. Tight glycemic control has been shown to decrease the risk of surgical site infection and to decrease mortality and the risk of infection in critically ill postoperative patients.

There have been no published studies of tight glycemic control in medical ICU or floor patients. Most experts would recommend keeping blood glucose (BG) at 90–180 mg/dL in general medical floor patients. In many intensive care and coronary care units, where patients are sicker and more closely monitored, the goal for glycemic control is even tighter: 80–110 mg/dL.

To effectively manage diabetes in the hospital, you need to know:

Does the patient have type 1 or type 2 diabetes?

Although all insulin-treated patients are likely to require insulin during acute illness, a type 1 patient *absolutely must* continue to receive insulin even if he or she is not eating, to prevent ketoacidosis.

What is the patient's outpatient medication regimen, and how effective was it prior to admission?

Will the patient be able to eat?

A Recommendation based on consistent and good quality patient-oriented evidence. **B** Recommendation based on inconsistent or limited quality patient-oriented evidence. **C** Recommendation based on usual practice, consensus, opinion, disease-oriented evidence, or case series for studies of diagnosis, treatment, and prevention of screening.

There have been few trials comparing inpatient management strategies for diabetes in general medical patients. These recommended orders are based primarily on clinical experience and expert opinion.

Patients Treated with Insulin

Example orders for a patient who is eating:
Insulin glargine 25 units SQ qhs
Insulin lispro 4 units SQ before breakfast, 6 units SQ before lunch and dinner
Correction dose insulin per algorithm for premeal hyperglycemia
Check capillary blood glucose (BG) qac and qhs

Insulin therapy for this patient has three components:

- *Basal insulin.* This is intermediate- or long-acting insulin; in this case, insulin glargine. If the patient is eating and has not had hypoglycemia, the patient's usual basal insulin dose should be prescribed.
- *Prandial insulin.* This is the rapid- or short-acting insulin given prior to meals, in this case insulin lispro. If the patient is eating and has not had hypoglycemia, the patient's usual prandial insulin dose should be prescribed.
- *Correction-dose insulin.* This is supplemental, rapid-acting insulin given prior to meals *in addition* to the usual prandial insulin to correct hyperglycemia. The rapid-acting insulins, insulin lispro and aspart, are ideal for correction doses because both their onset and offset are rapid. Correction doses should not be given more frequently than every 4 hours to prevent "stacking up" of doses and hypoglycemia.

The amount of insulin given as a correction dose depends on the usual insulin dose. Patients on relatively low doses of insulin, < 40 units per day, typically receive one additional unit of rapid-acting insulin for each 50 mg/dL that the BG is greater than 150 mg/dL. Patients on higher doses of insulin are more insulin resistant and require higher correction doses.

Suggested correction-dose insulin algorithms are shown in Table 1:

Table 1

Low-Dose Algorithm (for Patients on ≤ 40 Units of Insulin/Day)

Premeal BG	Additional Insulin Lispro
150–199	1 unit
200–249	2 units
250–299	3 units
300–349	4 units
> 349	5 units

Medium-Dose Algorithm (for Patients on 40–80 Units of Insulin/Day)

Premeal BG	Additional Insulin Lispro
150–199	1 unit
200–249	3 units
250–299	5 units
300–349	7 units
> 349	8 units

High-Dose Algorithm (for Patients on > 80 Units of Insulin/Day)

Premeal BG	Additional Insulin Lispro
150–199	2 units
200–249	4 units
250–299	7 units
300–349	10 units
> 349	12 units

BG, blood glucose.

Example Orders for a Patient Who Is Not Eating:

NPH insulin 15 units SQ q AM and qhs ($\frac{2}{3}$ of patient's home dose)
HOLD regular insulin
Check capillary BG q 6 hours
Correction-dose insulin per low-dose algorithm if BG > 180 mg/dL

There are two options for insulin-treated patients who are unable to eat:

- A continuous infusion of regular insulin ("insulin drip")
- Adjustment of the outpatient SQ insulin regimen

With appropriate training and very careful monitoring and adjustment, insulin drips are safe and effective. Insulin drips are commonly used to achieve tight glycemic control in the ICU and surgical settings but are sometimes not available on a general medical ward. An insulin drip is the treatment of choice for patients with type 1 diabetes who will be unable to eat for more than 1 day. An example insulin drip protocol is presented in the Trence, 2003 reference.

When adjusting the SQ insulin regimen, again consider the three components:

- The basal insulin should be decreased to two-thirds of the patient's outpatient dose to avoid hypoglycemia. An exception is the type 1 patient treated with insulin glargine, who should receive 100% of the usual dose.
- Prandial insulin should be withheld if the patient is not eating.
- Correction-dose rapid-acting insulin can be given if the BG exceeds the target range of 90–180 mg/dL. Doses should not be given more frequently than every 4 hours to avoid hypoglycemia. If repeated correction doses are needed and there has been no hypoglycemia, consider increasing the basal insulin dose.

Patients Treated with Oral Agents:

Example orders for a patient who is eating:
Rosiglitazone 4 mg PO qd
Discontinue metformin
Check capillary BG qac and qhs
For premeal hyperglycemia, administer correction dose insulin per low-dose algorithm

Oral diabetes regimens may also require adjustment in the hospital. Metformin should almost always be stopped on admission because it is contraindicated in renal insufficiency, heart failure, liver disease, and hypoxia due to the risk of lactic acidosis. It can be restarted when the patient is clinically stable and ready for discharge, provided no contraindications still exist.

The major side effect of sulfonylureas (glyburide, glimepiride) and meglitinides (repaglinide, nateglenide) is hypoglycemia. If the patient may not be able to eat normally because of diagnostic testing, surgery, or illness, these drugs should also be stopped. They can be continued if the patient is able to eat as usual.

The glitazones, rosiglitazone and pioglitazone, can cause sodium and fluid retention even in patients with normal left ventricular function. They are contraindicated in patients with New York Heart Association (NYHA) Class III or IV heart failure and should be used with careful monitoring in patients with other cardiovascular disease.

Premeal hyperglycemia can be treated with correction-dose rapid-acting insulin.

Example Orders for a Patient Who Is Not Eating:

Discontinue glyburide and metformin
Check capillary BG q 6 hours, and call if > 180 mg/dL

All oral agents should be discontinued and resumed when the patient is able to eat. Capillary BG should be measured at least four times daily.

Depending on the severity of illness, some patients may have normal BG while NPO and off oral diabetes medications. More severely stressed patients are likely to become hyperglycemic. For an ICU patient with a BG goal of 80–110 mg/dL, an insulin infusion may be needed. In floor patients, correction-dose insulin can be ordered if BG exceeds

180 mg/dL. If correction-dose insulin is actually required, begin a conservative dose of an intermediate or long-acting insulin, adjusting as necessary to keep BG in the goal range.

References

Clement S, Braithwaite SS, Magee MF, et al: Management of diabetes and hyperglycemia in hospitals. *Diabetes Care* 27:553–591, 2004.

Trence DL, Kelly JL, Hirsch IB: The rationale and management for inpatients with cardiovascular disease: time for a change. *JCEM* 88:2430–2437, 2003.

Acute Pain Management

Pain is very common in hospitalized patients, regardless of the primary diagnosis. Effective pain control can lead to earlier discharge, avoid complications, and improve the patient's experience of hospitalization. When treating pain, follow these steps:

1. Assess and document pain intensity, location, and quality.
2. Evaluate response to treatment at regular intervals.
3. Individualize the treatment regimen with respect to agent, dose, route, and frequency.
4. Administer analgesics on schedule if pain is persistent.
5. Recognize side effects of treatment and manage as necessary.

Nonopioid Analgesics

Acetaminophen and nonsteroidal anti-inflammatory drugs (NSAIDs) may be used alone to treat mild pain and some forms of moderate pain.

Table 2 Dosing Recommendations for Commonly Used Nonopioid Analgesics for Pain*

Agent	Initial Dosing for Pain	Comments
Acetaminophen	650 mg PO/PR q 4–6 h	NTE 4 g/day; limit to < 2 g/day in patients with liver disease
Aspirin	325–650 mg PO/ PR q 4–6 h	NTE 4 g/day; anti-inflammatory effects with plasma levels of 150–300 µg/mL
Ibuprofen	400 mg PO q 4–6 h	
Naproxen	500 mg initially, then 250 mg PO q 6–8 h	
Ketorolac	30–60 mg IV/IM initially, then 15–30 mg IV/IM q 6 h	NTE 5 days due to increased risk of GI bleed

*This table is not all inclusive.
PR, per rectum; NTE, not to exceed.

Acetaminophen and NSAIDs may also be used for more severe pain in combination with opioids to provide an opioid dose-sparing effect.

Avoid NSAIDs in patients with renal disease, end-stage liver disease, peptic ulcer disease, coagulopathies, and heart failure and in those with a history of hypersensitivity to aspirin or other NSAIDs.

There are no published data demonstrating that a particular NSAID provides more pain relief than another (Table 2).

Opioid Analgesics

Opioids should be used to treat moderate to severe pain.

Patients vary greatly in their analgesic dose requirements and responses to opioid analgesics. Reassess patients frequently to evaluate the efficacy of the current regimen and adjust as necessary.

Fentanyl, meperidine, and methadone are the *least* likely opioids to induce an allergic response in a patient with a history of an allergic reaction (generalized rash, shortness of breath) to either codeine or morphine

Avoid opioids in patients with acute or severe bronchial asthma, paralytic ileus or gastrointestinal (GI) obstruction, and respiratory depression (Tables 3 and 4).

Managing Opioid Side Effects

- *Constipation*: Stool softener plus a laxative (docusate + senna, bisacodyl, milk of magnesia, etc.)
- *Itching*: Antihistamine (diphenhydramine, hydroxyzine, cetirizine, etc.) ± switching opioid analgesics
- *Nausea*: Tolerance often develops rapidly. Use an antiemetic as needed (prochlorperazine, promethazine, metoclopramide, ondansetron, etc.)
- *Sedation*: Hold opioid analgesic and other central nervous system (CNS) depressants or decrease dose. Evaluate other potential causes and use naloxone as necessary if accompanied by respiratory depression

References

Carr DB, Jacox AK, Chapman CR, et al: Acute Pain Management: Operative or Medical Procedures and Trauma. Clinical Practice. Guideline No. 1. AHCPR Publication No. 92-0032. Rockville, MD: Agency for Healthcare Policy and Research, Public Health Service, U.S. Department of Health and Human Services, 1992.

Li JM: Pain management in the hospitalized patient. *Med Clin North Am* 86:1–21, 2002.

Table 3 Dosing Recommendations for Commonly Used Opioids for Pain*

Agent	Typical Starting Dose	Indication	Comments
Morphine	2–10 mg IV/IM/SQ q 3–4 h or 15–30 mg PO q 3–6 h	Severe pain	Active metabolite may accumulate in setting of renal failure
Morphine controlled-release	15–30 mg PO q 8–12 h	Severe pain that is persistent or chronic	Dosage must be individualized
Oxycodone	5–15 mg PO q 3–4 h	Moderate to severe pain	
Oxycodone controlled-release	10–20 mg PO q 12 h	Severe pain that is persistent or chronic	Dosage must be individualized
Hydromorphone	0.5–2 mg IV/IM/SQ q 3–4 h or 2–8 mg PO q 3–4 h	Severe pain	
Fentanyl	25–100 μg IV q 1–2 h	Sedation and procedural pain	Buccal lozenge also available
Meperidine	25–100 mg IV/IM/SQ q 3–4 h	Moderate to severe pain	Limit use < 48 hours and < 600 mg/day; avoid if CrCl < 30 mL/min
Methadone	2.5–10 mg IV/IM q 4–8 h or 5–20 mg PO q 4–8 h	Severe pain	May accumulate in adipose tissue and cause delayed toxicity

*There are unpredictable degrees of incomplete cross-tolerance to various opioid effects among agents (analgesia and adverse effects). Trials with multiple agents may be necessary to obtain optimal efficacy and tolerability. Increase the dose if relief is inadequate and change the frequency if duration of action is insufficient.
CrCl, creatinine clearance.

Table 4 Equianalgesic Interchange (Approximate)

Agent	IV/IM/SQ	Oral
Morphine	10 mg	30 mg
Oxycodone	N/A	20 mg
Hydromorphone	1.5 mg	7.5 mg
Methadone	1–10 mg	2–20 mg
Fentanyl	0.1 mg	N/A (actiq = buccal)
Meperidine	75 mg	300 mg

N/A, not available.

Max MB, Payne R, Edwards WT, et al: *Principles of Analgesic Use in the Treatment of Acute Pain and Cancer Pain,* ed 4. Glenview, IL: American Pain Society, 1999.

Comfort Care

In the setting of life-limiting illness, comfort care strives to provide the patient and family with treatment that relieves the patient's distressful symptoms and responds to patient and family psychological, social, emotional, and spiritual concerns. Comfort care should be initiated only after discussion with and agreement by the patient or surrogate decision-maker.

Admit to: Floor

In many circumstances, comfort care can be provided for patients at home via hospice or in skilled nursing facilities.

Diagnosis: Comfort Care

Condition: Serious

Vital Signs:

Prn only if needed to enhance patient comfort
If vital signs (VS) will not be used to guide intervention or therapy, do not do them.

Allergies: Routine

Activity: As Tolerated

Consider positioning changes to prevent painful skin breakdown and to maximize comfort.

Nursing:

Oxygen 0–6 L/min nasal cannula prn dyspnea. Titrate to patient comfort
Suction only for severe throat secretions
Oral care q 2 hours and prn
Foley catheter or condom catheter prn for patient comfort

Diet: As Tolerated

IV Fluids: None

IV fluids (IVF) can contribute to pulmonary edema and anasarca. In rare circumstances, IVF may improve patient comfort. However, in most cases, IVF should not be given.

The introduction of IV lines should be kept to a minimum.

Medications:

Morphine sulfate immediate release 10–30 mg PO/sublingual (SL) q 2 hours prn pain,

or morphine sulfate 1–2 mg IV q 1 hour prn pain,
or morphine sulfate continuous IV infusion at 1–2 mg/h

For inadequate pain relief with continuous infusion, bolus with dose equal to current hourly rate and increase infusion by 25–50% q 30 minutes prn pain

Notify MD if inadequate pain relief after 4 bolus doses and dose titrations

Tylenol 650 mg PO/per rectum (PR) q 4–6 hours prn pain or fever

Lorazepam 0.5–1 mg PO/SL/IV q 1 hour prn anxiety/restlessness/dyspnea

Scopolamine patch 1.5 mg topically to mastoid q 72 hours prn secretions

Atropine 0.4 mg SQ q 3 hours prn secretions

Milk of magnesium 30 mL PO bid prn constipation

Bisacodyl suppository 1 PR qd prn constipation

Docusate 250 mg PO bid for any patient on narcotics. Hold for loose stool

Senna 2 tablets PO bid for any patient on narcotics. Hold for loose stool

Diphenoxylate/atropine (Lomotil) 1–2 tablets PO q 4 hours prn diarrhea. Limit 8 tablets/24 hours

Metoclopramide 10 mg PO/IV q 4 hours prn nausea

Promethazine 12.5–25 mg PO/IV q 4 hours prn nausea

Prochlorperazine 25 mg suppository PR q 8 hours prn nausea

Diphenhydramine 25–50 mg PO/IV q 6 hours prn itching or insomnia

Zolpidem 5–10 mg PO qhs prn insomnia

Dextromethorphan 15–30 mg PO qid prn cough

Benzonatate 100 mg PO qid prn cough

The opioid and benzodiazepine doses listed here are recommendations for average-weight adults who are opioid and benzodiazepine naïve. The doses of opioids and benzodiazepines needed to relieve symptoms without causing burdensome side effects will vary based on several patient factors such as age, weight, renal function, and prior exposure to opioids or benzodiazepines. ●

Medications that add to a patient's comfort should be continued or initiated. Medications that are not necessary for comfort should be discontinued. ●

Labs and Diagnostic Studies:

None

Discharge Planning:

Consider hospice referral and/or nursing home placement if the patient and family would like to have the patient's care transitioned to outside of the hospital.

Special Considerations:

Please make sure that a do not attempt resuscitation order is completed
Consult social work. Consider spiritual care consultation.

Reference

Storey P, Knight C, Schonwetter RS: *Hospice/Palliative Care Training for Physicians: Pocket Guide to Hospice/Palliative Medicine.* Glenview, IL: American Academy of Hospice and Palliative Medicine, 2003.

Transfusion

Patients with symptomatic anemia without active bleeding may require admission for urgent transfusion. There is no universal hematocrit threshold for transfusion—the decision to transfuse should be based on the patient's symptoms, co-morbid illness, and severity of anemia. In general, an otherwise healthy adult should not be transfused unless the hematocrit is

< 21% *or* he or she has significant symptoms and is unlikely to respond to specific therapy for anemia (i.e., iron, folate, erythropoietin [EPO]) within a reasonable time frame.

Transfusion may be indicated for patients with hematocrit 21–30% and cardiac or respiratory disease or other acute illness. Transfusion is not indicated for patients with hematocrit > 30% unless actively bleeding.

Patients should be counseled on the risks and benefits of transfusion and should explicitly consent to the procedure. Current estimates of risk of transmission of viral infection per unit transfused are:

- HIV: < 1 in 1.9 million
- Hepatitis C virus (HCV): < 1 in 1 million
- Hepatitis B virus (HBV): 1 in 1 million
- Human T-cell lymphotropic virus (HTLV) I and II: 1:164,000

These orders are for a 72-year-old man with myelodysplasia admitted with severe anemia and dyspnea limiting his ability to care for himself at home.

Admit to: Observation Unit

The hospital location depends on the severity of symptoms and anemia. Most stable patients can be transfused in an infusion center or observation unit. Patients with more severe symptoms and those requiring multiple units of blood may be admitted to the medical ward, or in cases of cardiac ischemia, the ICU.

Diagnosis: Transfusion

Condition: Stable

Vital Signs:

Routine, with VS q 15 minutes during transfusion. Stop transfusion and call house officer (HO) for fever, tachycardia, or hypotension

Frequent VS are done to allow early detection of transfusion reactions. The transfusion should be stopped whenever a transfusion reaction is suspected.

Acute hemolytic transfusion reactions are a life-threatening emergency and present with fever; hypotension; tachycardia; dyspnea; chest, back or flank pain; nausea; anxiety; and/or hemoglobinuria.

Febrile nonhemolytic transfusion reactions are both more common and more benign and are caused by recipient reaction to donor leukocytes and cytokines. Patients develop fever during transfusion but have no other signs or symptoms.

Fever may also herald bacterial contamination of blood products.

Transfusion-related acute lung injury presents with dyspnea, hypoxia, hypotension, fever, and diffuse pulmonary infiltrates, during or up to 6 hours after transfusion.

Urticarial or allergic reactions are the most common complication of transfusion. Most patients simply have itching or hives. Rare patients have full-blown anaphylaxis with shock and angioedema, which can occur within minutes. Most of these patients have IgA deficiency and should be tested in case future transfusion is required.

Allergies: NKDA

Activity: Ad Lib

Patients with severe anemia and cardiac symptoms should limit activity until after transfusion.

Nursing:

Type and cross 2 units of packed red blood cells, and transfuse each over 2 hours

The rate of transfusion depends on the severity of symptoms and the patient's risk of volume overload with blood administration. A patient with severe symptomatic anemia and chest pain may receive the transfusion more quickly, whereas a stable patient with known heart failure may receive it more slowly.

Blood products may need modification or special screening for certain patient populations:

- **Cytomegalovirus (CMV)-negative blood products** should be used for CMV-negative patients who are, or will be, severely immunosuppressed. This includes patients who have had or will have solid organ or bone marrow transplants and HIV-positive patients.
- **Leukocyte-reduced blood products** may prevent alloimmunization, febrile nonhemolytic transfusion reactions, and transmission of CMV. Leukocyte-reduced products should be ordered for patients having bone marrow and some solid organ transplants, those with a history of febrile transfusion reactions, and those for whom CMV-negative products are indicated but not available.
- **Gamma-irradiated blood products** should be used for patients having bone marrow transplant or aggressive chemotherapy and those with any lymphoproliferative malignancy, to kill all leukocytes and prevent graft versus host disease.

Diet: Regular

IV Fluids: None

Each unit of packed red blood cells is about 350 mL. IVF are usually not given along with blood unless the patient is actively bleeding.

M edications:

Diphenhydramine 25–50 mg IV or PO prn itching or urticaria
Acetaminophen 650 mg PO q 6 hours prn fever or pain

Routine premedication is not indicated for all patients having transfusion.

Diphenhydramine can prevent or treat urticarial reactions, which are relatively common and are due to allergy to the blood donor's serum proteins. Diphenhydramine should be given before transfusion to patients who have had this reaction in the past. Corticosteroids (hydrocortisone 100 mg IV prior to transfusion) may also be effective.

Acetaminophen can be used to treat febrile nonhemolytic transfusion reactions.

Drugs that should be prescribed for specific causes of anemia include:

1. EPO or darbopoietin for kidney disease, HIV, or chemotherapy-related anemia
2. Iron for iron deficiency, administered with vitamin C or orange juice to improve absorption.
3. Vitamin B_{12} for B_{12} deficiency, administered either daily PO or monthly IM
4. Folate for folate deficiency
5. Immunosuppressive medications for autoimmune hemolytic anemia

L abs and Diagnostic Studies:

Post-transfusion hematocrit

The hematocrit should rise by 3–4% for every unit of blood transfused to a 70-kg patient.

Of course, more extensive laboratory evaluation is indicated for patients with an undiagnosed cause of anemia.

GI endoscopy should be considered in any patient with unexplained iron-deficiency anemia to exclude GI sources of blood loss, including malignant lesions.

Discharge Planning:

Most patients without active bleeding will be able to go home after a very short hospital stay. Discharge education should focus on:

- Close follow-up for early detection of recurrent anemia so that future transfusions may be performed in a more elective, outpatient setting
- Dietary recommendations for patients with nutritional deficiencies
- Pharmacy review of prescribed medications

Special Considerations:

Patients should be monitored closely, and the transfusion should be stopped immediately if there is any sign of transfusion reaction.

If an acute hemolytic transfusion reaction is suspected:

- Stop the transfusion.
- Check and support the ABCs—airway, breathing, circulation.
- Start isotonic fluid at 250 mL/h to initiate diuresis.
- Check the blood bag—the majority of hemolytic transfusion reactions are still caused by clerical error.
- Send the following labs: free serum hemoglobin, direct antibody (Coombs) test, urine hemoglobin, and repeat

crossmatch. (Some hospitals also centrifuge a sample of blood—if the serum has a pink tinge, substantial hemolysis has occurred.)

■ Call your hospital's blood bank for further recommendations on evaluation and management.

If a patient has fever but no other signs or symptoms, the diagnosis is likely febrile nonhemolytic transfusion reaction. The unit of blood should be discarded, and future transfusions should be with leukocyte-reduced blood and preadministration of acetaminophen.

Patients with itching or urticaria should receive diphenhydramine. If they improve and have no other signs or symptoms, the transfusion may be resumed.

Reference

Puget Sound Blood Center Blood Component Reference Manual: www.psbc.org/bcrm/index.htm; accessed 12/5/05.
Contact your local blood center for specific recommendations for your area.

Venous Thromboembolism Prophylaxis

Venous thromboembolism (VTE) is common in hospitalized patients, and its first clinical manifestation may be death—pulmonary embolism causes 10% of deaths in U.S. hospitals. Without prophylaxis, symptomatic and asymptomatic VTE will develop in 10–20% of medical patients and an even larger proportion of surgical and ICU patients.

Risk factors for VTE in medical patients include:

■ Congestive heart failure, especially NYHA Class III and IV
■ Chronic obstructive pulmonary disease (COPD) exacerbation

- Sepsis
- History of VTE
- Advanced age
- Stroke with lower-extremity weakness
- Cancer
- Inflammatory bowel disease
- Obesity
- Central line

Patients with heart failure or respiratory illness and those confined to bed with one or more risk factors for VTE should receive prophylaxis. Options for prophylaxis include:

- Heparin 5000 units SQ q 8 hours **Ⓐ**
- Enoxaparin 30 mg SQ q 24 hours **Ⓐ**
- Compression stockings and sequential compression devices **Ⓑ** for patients with contraindications to pharmacologic prophylaxis (active bleeding, epidural catheter, history of heparin-induced thrombocytopenia)

Reference

Geerts WH, Pineo GF, Heit JA, et al: Prevention of venous thromboembolism: The Seventh ACCP Consensus Conference on Antithrombotic and Thrombolytic Therapy. *Chest* 126:338S–400S, 2004.

Index

Page numbers followed by t indicate tables.